MINDFULNESS WORKBOOK
FOR STRESS RELIEF

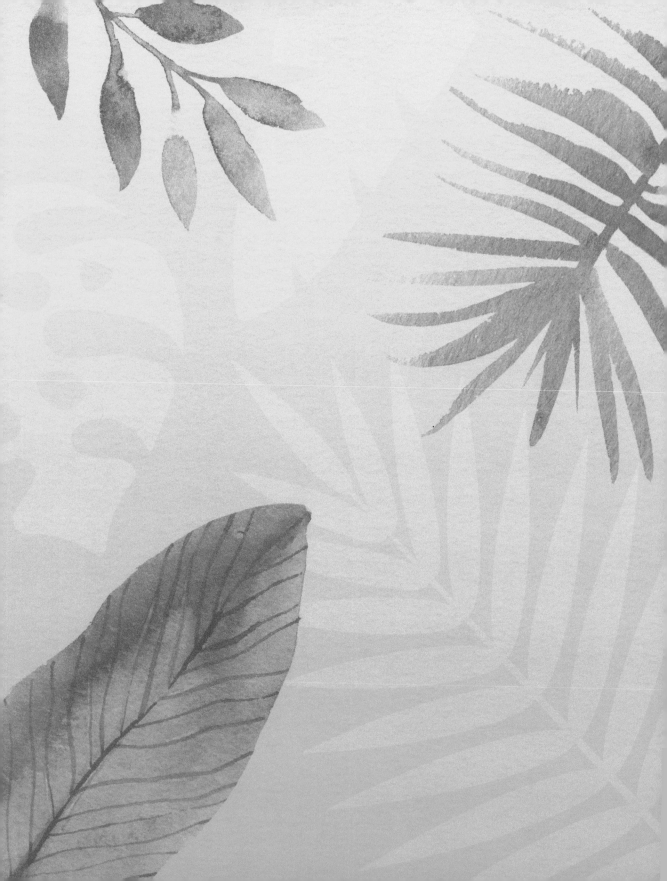

Mindfulness Workbook for
STRESS RELIEF

REDUCE STRESS *through Meditation, Non-Judgment,
Mind-Body Awareness, and Self-Inquiry*

APRIL SNOW, LMFT

ROCKRIDGE
PRESS

For general information on our other products and services or to obtain technical support, please contact our Customer Care Department within the United States at (866) 744-2665, or outside the United States at (510) 253-0500.

Rockridge Press publishes its books in a variety of electronic and print formats. Some content that appears in print may not be available in electronic books, and vice versa.

Interior and Cover Designer: Brian Lewis
Art Producer: Samantha Ulban
Editor: Vanessa Ta
Production Editor: Rachel Taenzler

Illustrations © 2020 Julia Kretschmann. All other images used under license iStock and Shutterstock. Author photo courtesy of Lauren Selfridge and Tristan Brand Photography.

ISBN: Print 978-1-64739-804-0
eBook 978-1-64739-923-8
R0

To Grandmom, my first mindfulness teacher, who always reminds me to "be in the moment."

CONTENTS

INTRODUCTION

If you picked up this book, you are most likely experiencing stress in your life right now. Chronic stress can wreak havoc on your physical and emotional well-being, often leading to anxiety, depression, irritability, difficulty concentrating, insomnia, digestive issues, headaches, or chronic pain. Left unchecked, stress can impact every area of your life, such as your ability to perform at work, communicate clearly, or take care of your basic needs.

If stress is so destructive, why does society tell you to push ahead during difficult times? Sitting with the discomfort of stress is challenging, but as you'll learn in this book, being more aware is actually the key to decreasing stress, chronic pain, and uncomfortable emotions.

Mindfulness allows you to release judgments about what you should be doing, let go of comparison, and be present in your life moment to moment. Instead of running away from what's causing you stress, you can begin to understand why you're feeling stressed and what you can do to feel relaxed again. By slowing down to practice the meditations and exercises in this book, you will begin to know yourself on a deeper level and understand what your body needs to feel balanced and calm. You may be surprised just how accessible, simple, and effective mindfulness can be. It's not all twisty yoga poses and sitting perfectly still with a clear mind; you can incorporate mindfulness into everyday experiences such as sitting, walking, or eating.

For the past 20 years, mindfulness has been my most dependable and consistent source of support. There were many years where I existed in survival mode, cycling in and out of depression and anxiety and feeling disconnected from myself. During my early years in college, I discovered yoga and mindfulness, which began my journey of slowly reconnecting to myself. I weaved in and out of my mindfulness practice throughout my 20s until I had a wake-up call that showed me exactly how powerful mindfulness can be in times of distress.

Grieving a relationship loss and feeling extremely burned out at work, I entered into a deep depression and found myself in therapy for the first time. Therapy helped get me back on my feet, but there was something missing. In my search for a deeper understanding of myself, I took a sabbatical from work to travel to India and fully immerse myself in meditation and yoga. Doing so allowed me to step out of my need to work so much and be a people-pleaser. While away, I was able to meditate and practice yoga every day for a month. Afterward, I was shocked by how resilient I felt and how well I was able to effortlessly manage some big stressors that came up while traveling back home.

When I returned home I continued my mindfulness practice, and about two years later, I moved to California to pursue my master's degree in psychology at the California Institute of Integral Studies. During my training, I was introduced to mindfulness-based stress reduction (MBSR), and I eventually started teaching mindfulness workshops and incorporating mindfulness into my work with my therapy clients. Since then, I have led self-care retreats, clinical trainings, and therapy groups, all using mindfulness tools. I am still amazed at the power of mindfulness to calm a stressed-out nervous system or to help someone access insights that were out of reach through talk alone.

Thankfully, you don't need to take a sabbatical, go on a retreat, or commit to any type of spiritual ideology to start your own mindfulness practice. Although mindfulness was born out of Buddhist meditation, it has become a widely used secular practice. A significant contributor to the popularity and accessibility of mindfulness has been the MBSR program originally developed by Jon Kabat-Zinn at the University of Massachusetts Medical Center over 40 years ago. This book will help you discover the foundational practices of MBSR, which have been proven to reduce the effects of stress. You'll come away from this book with a road map for designing your own mindfulness practice, a better understanding of yourself, and specific tools to help you reduce stress throughout many areas of your life.

HOW TO USE THIS WORKBOOK

This workbook is an introduction to the practices of mindfulness-based stress reduction (MBSR) and offers a wide variety of practical mindfulness tools to add to your self-care toolbox. Not only will you discover why mindfulness is such a powerful stress reliever, but you'll also learn exercises to help you reduce stress in many areas of life.

In the first two chapters, you'll be introduced to the foundational practices of MBSR, such as seated meditation, body scan, breath awareness, and mindful walking, as well as informal practices to bring a sense of mindful awareness to everyday moments. These exercises will form the base of your mindfulness practice going forward and are proven tools to reduce stress stemming from many causes. Chapter 3 will use these practices to relieve stress in your relationships, and chapter 4 will address stress at work. In chapter 5, you'll begin to deepen your mindful self-care practice with gentle yoga postures, self-compassion exercises, and instructions for organizing an entire day of mindfulness. Finally, chapter 6 will help you use these practices to manage challenges such as anxiety, chronic pain, and sleep issues.

As you devote more energy to your mindfulness practice and begin to increase self-awareness, you may begin to notice deeper wounds, memories, or other stressors emerging. Chapters 5 and 6 will guide you through these roadblocks, which may include an inability to sit in silence, a tough inner critic, managing uncomfortable emotions including anxiety and depression, or sitting with grief after a loss. If at any point you become overwhelmed by the thoughts and feelings surfacing during your practice, I encourage you to seek out the support of a trained therapist or consult with your doctor.

Although each has a different focus, every chapter explores and provides guidance for practicing meditation, non-judgment, mind-body awareness, and self-inquiry. You can progress through the sections and exercises from start to finish, or jump ahead into a specific section based on your interests and current areas of stress. For instance, you may be experiencing tension in your relationship and decide to jump immediately to chapter 3 to practice the Mindful Listening exercise (page 62) with your significant other. Or perhaps you've had a mindfulness practice for quite some time and want to dive immediately into the emotional self-inquiry work of chapter 5.

No matter which approach you take, give yourself time to move through this workbook. Keep in mind that traditional MBSR programs are eight weeks long and include a full day of mindfulness, but even that is just the beginning of creating a personal mindfulness practice. You will have the most success by taking a quality over quantity approach. Pick one or two of the formal MBSR exercises from chapter 1 to focus on each week, sprinkling in a few of the others as you go. For the best results, slowly build up your mindfulness routine to practice most days of the week for at least 10 minutes per day, or 25 to 30 minutes for optimal stress-reduction benefits.

When you're ready to take your mindfulness practice and self-inquiry work even further, you will find additional resources and suggested reading materials at the end of the book (see page 170). You can also find audio recordings of many of the meditations and exercises in this book at my website, AprilSnowConsulting.com/stress-workbook.

01

Mindfulness and Stress

Mindfulness is a powerful and proven method of reducing stress and its negative health effects. A daily practice can help you feel calmer and gain clarity about yourself and what's happening in your life, like fog clearing after a storm. As you'll learn in this chapter, a significant number of health issues are stress-related. One particular mindfulness program, mindfulness-based stress reduction (MBSR), has been studied extensively and proven not only to minimize stress, but also to create lasting changes in your brain that improve your mental health and physical well-being. MBSR consists of a mixture of sitting and movement meditation exercises that you can customize to create a daily practice that meets your needs. In this chapter, you'll look more deeply into what mindfulness is and how to begin integrating these beneficial MBSR practices into your daily life.

WHY MINDFULNESS?

You may be hoping that mindfulness could be the solution to help you manage the stress, anxiety, or chronic pain you have been feeling but unsure why it would be different than any other self-care practice you've tried. It's true that mindfulness does help create a relaxation response in your body, but there's much more happening behind the scenes. Let's take a deeper look at how mindfulness can affect your brain and nervous system to help you manage stress levels and positively impact your overall physical and mental well-being.

When you're under stress, your prefrontal cortex at the front of your skull (which controls decision-making, emotional regulation, and empathy) shuts down, and your reptilian brain at the back of your skull takes over. The reptilian brain is the oldest part of your brain, which controls basic functions such as breathing and pumping blood. Being in this primitive state impacts how you are able to function at work and in your relationships. Practicing mindfulness helps keep your prefrontal cortex online, allowing you to feel more empathetic and compassionate in your relationships (Chiesa & Serretti, 2009) and more focused and productive at work (Good et al., 2015).

A huge component of any mindfulness practice is awareness of the breath. When you slow down your breath, especially elongating the exhale, you activate your parasympathetic nervous system, which is also known as the "rest-and-digest" component of your autonomic nervous system. Think of this state as the opposite of being in "fight-flight-freeze" mode, when your body is preparing to respond to a real or perceived threat by fighting off the danger, running away, or freezing in place. When your rest-and-digest system is engaged, you feel safe, relaxed, and focused. Your body is operating optimally, which is in contrast to fight-flight-freeze, when your body is literally in survival mode. Using mindful breathing can deactivate the stress response and help you step out of the discomfort of fight-flight-freeze.

The immediate effect of slowing down to breathe, practicing mindfulness, and being more present in our moment-to-moment experience is feeling more physically relaxed. Over time, however, the brain actually starts to change. This ability of the brain to rewire itself is called neuroplasticity, which research and brain scans have repeatedly shown occurs during meditation and mindfulness practices (Tolahunase et al., 2018).

I like to use the metaphor of a sponge. When you engage in mindfulness activities such as meditation or breathing exercises, you wring out your emotional sponge, which has become saturated with the stress, anxiety, and exhaustion of your busy life. This gives you more capacity to regulate your emotions and absorb stress. Thus, practicing mindfulness on a regular basis can literally restructure your brain to be less reactive to emotional triggers and more resilient to the impact of everyday stressors.

When your stress levels are lower and your brain is able to manage your emotions with ease, your overall mental health improves. Research has shown that MBSR reduces symptoms and lowers the recurrence of depression and anxiety for people who practice regularly, even for just a few minutes each day (Hoge et al., 2017). I often see this transformation in my psychotherapy work. Clients come into my office for the first time clearly exhausted, often from working too many hours or managing caregiver responsibilities. Their bodies tell me the whole story, as their shoulders are hunched over and their heads hang heavy. Sometimes clients will feel so lousy that they immediately collapse onto the couch when feeling depressed, or their eyes dart around the office when they're feeling anxious. As we begin to practice mindfulness together, after a few deep breaths or some gentle stretches in the office and following instructions for practicing at home, they become calmer and more balanced. Sometimes this change happens quickly, in just a few weeks; other times it takes a few months, depending on the severity of stress in their lives.

THE MIND-BODY CONNECTION

Although you may not have noticed the correlation, when under stress for an extended period of time, you're more likely to get sick, experience digestive problems, or have flare-ups of other health conditions, such as psoriasis or chronic pain. According to a nationwide study, up to 80 percent of medical visits involve a stress-related component, which can include everything from high blood pressure, constipation, allergies, and headaches to anxiety and depression (Nerurkar et al., 2013; Harvard Medical

School, n.d.). When you're in a heightened state of stress, whether from a real or perceived threat, your nervous system goes into fight-flight-freeze mode, forcing important bodily systems offline in preparation for survival. Your body isn't able to operate at full capacity under prolonged duress, and you may get physically and/or mentally ill as a result.

I always know I have been pushing myself too hard when I wake up with a sore throat or my skin begins to show inflammation. My body is sending me the message to slow down and pay attention to my needs. When I start to feel this way, my mood immediately begins to match my physical state. I become more irritable, anxious, and pessimistic when I'm not feeling well, and I just want to hide from the world (and myself).

On the flip side, when I'm incorporating yoga and mindfulness into my routine on a regular basis, I feel much more resilient to stress. It always amazes me just how little I feel bothered by things, if I do at all, when I'm practicing meditation or just paying more attention to my moment-to-moment experience. Even if I don't feel perfect, my mood stays positive rather than catastrophizing about what could go wrong. Apparently I'm not alone in seeing this correlation, as studies have shown that MBSR actually increases your capacity for self-compassion and decreases rumination, otherwise known as obsessive thinking (Sevinc et al., 2018).

Have you also become aware of how your body and mind (thoughts, emotions, beliefs) seem to influence each other? You can harness this ability to decrease stress and increase your overall well-being on a physical and emotional level. Countless research studies have shown the positive effects of practicing MBSR for reducing a wide range of stress-related symptoms such as anxiety and depression (Kabat-Zinn et al., 1992) and chronic pain (Kabat-Zinn et al., 1985).

A huge component of the mind-body connection is the ability of mind-fulness to literally change your brain, increasing neuroplasticity in eight different regions (Stahl & Goldstein, 2019). Studies conducted by Sara Lazar, PhD, a researcher at Massachusetts General Hospital and professor at Harvard Medical School, showed that meditation practitioners under-going an eight-week MBSR program displayed increased thickness in areas of the prefrontal cortex that aid memory, learning, decision-making, atten-tion, sensory processing, and body awareness. Even more exciting is that these changes were most noticeable in older participants, indicating that mindfulness practice could potentially reverse the effects of age-related thinning in these sections of the brain (Lazar et al., 2005).

Practicing mindfulness helps you become aware of the stress in your life and the effect it has on your body and emotional state. By tuning in to the present moment, you can start to create a relationship with your experience and understand that there are layers beyond the stress, pain, or illness. You can also begin to see your strengths, unmet needs, and what choices you can make to care for yourself. For instance, if you're constantly feeling anxious, you may find it difficult to concentrate on your work or get enough sleep. When you start to reflect on the underlying cause of your anxiety, you may realize that you're sensitive to caffeine or that you need to set more boundaries on your availability at work.

Overall, research has shown that practicing MBSR for just eight weeks, for an average of 27 minutes per day, can have a significant impact on your overall well-being and emotional regulation (Holzel et al., 2011). Not only can you decrease your stress and anxiety levels by calming the fight-flight-freeze response, but you can also become more self-aware and empathetic toward others. Practicing mindfulness on a consistent basis can have a positive effect on so many aspects of your life.

WHAT EXACTLY IS MINDFULNESS?

Now that you've learned more about the benefits of mindfulness for stress, you are probably curious about what the actual practice entails. Perhaps you imagine long sessions on a meditation cushion while cultivating a clear, empty mind or reaching a state of internal peace. Whether you're new to mindfulness or have been practicing for some time, that can feel daunting to achieve. In our busy, fast-paced lives, it is becoming increasingly difficult to slow down, and when we do, the reverberating noise can be uncomfortable to sit with. Do you ever notice that the more tired you are, the more difficult it is to sit with yourself or fall asleep? Ironically, the more you need quiet and rest, the harder they are to access.

In reality, mindfulness is much simpler and more accessible than trying to achieve perfect stillness or a mind clear of distracting thoughts or worries. According to Jon Kabat-Zinn, mindfulness is simply the awareness that you experience when you pay attention, on purpose and without judgment, to the present moment (Kabat-Zinn, 2013). Mindfulness from an MBSR perspective can be practiced both formally and informally. Formal practice is a bit more structured, such as sitting in meditation or doing a series of yoga postures, whereas informal practice is simply noticing and embracing whatever is present as you engage with yourself, your daily activities, your surroundings, or others. Instead of disavowing your busy mind or disconnecting from the world, you can bring awareness and acceptance to the complexity of your experiences.

The beauty of mindfulness is that it can be practiced in any moment, wherever you are. For instance, you can mindfully observe the pace of your breath during a work meeting or slowly eat your breakfast, noticing the textures and tastes of each bite. You can also be mindful when walking your dog as you take in the blue sky and cool breeze on your skin. When you stand in line at the grocery store, try feeling your feet on the ground and noting your thoughts.

Why is being with the present moment so important? When you get stuck worrying about the past or stressing about the "what-ifs" of the future, not only do you miss out on your life, but you also create unnecessary stress on your body. You miss those little joys and get sick more often. Focusing on the here and now helps you feel calmer and more grounded in reality.

In the sections that follow, you'll explore some of the main components of mindfulness: meditation, non-judgment, mind-body awareness, self-inquiry, and practice. Throughout the book, you'll revisit these components through different lenses to enable you to practice mindfulness in every area of your life, such as in your relationships and at work.

Meditation

If you're practicing mindfulness anytime you bring awareness without judgment to your present experience, what is meditation? To differentiate meditation from mindfulness, think of meditation as one part of your overall mindfulness practice. During meditation, you intentionally set aside time to still the body and focus the mind on your internal experience, whereas everyday mindfulness is somewhat spontaneous and includes more engagement with your external experience. I find it helpful to put these two practices through the MBSR lens, where meditation can be labeled as a more formal, structured practice that includes time set aside for seated or movement practices on a daily basis.

What's confusing is that mindfulness and meditation can look very similar on the outside. For example, let's look at seated mindfulness versus meditation. You might be sitting quietly in a chair in the waiting room of your doctor's office. Instead of looking at your phone or a magazine, you decide to mindfully observe your thoughts, emotions, and physical sensations while you wait to be called. In this moment, you are practicing mindfulness while still being slightly engaged in your external environment. Meditation, on the other hand, would involve going inward to focus solely on your breath and internal experience.

If you're practicing mindfulness throughout the day, you may wonder why you need a formal meditation practice. Mindfulness alone doesn't necessarily create the same levels of neurological change, emotional resilience, or self-awareness that have been shown to result from a consistent MBSR practice. I see meditation as the path to creating a deeper understanding of yourself. Instead of just managing stress and anxiety when it surfaces, you can go even further into your awareness to understand what needs aren't being met or what emotions you're feeling. That awareness allows you to create more lasting change in your life so that you experience less stress and anxiety overall. Think of it as a doctor uncovering the source of a symptom, not just putting a bandage on top.

If you are new to meditation or MBSR, you may be wondering what the formal practice looks like or what props you might need. Next, you'll find the steps to practice a Simple Seated Meditation, showing just how straightforward it is to get started. At the end of this chapter, you'll find more simple meditations you can incorporate into your daily mindfulness routine.

SIMPLE SEATED MEDITATION

You can do this meditation anywhere: sitting on the floor, on a chair, under a tree, in your car, or even at your desk at work. An audio recording of this meditation is available at AprilSnowConsulting.com/stress-workbook.

1. Find a quiet spot to sit still for five minutes without interruption. It can be helpful to set a timer when first getting started to ease any anxiety about keeping track of time.

2. Sit comfortably in a straight-backed chair with feet on the floor, or cross-legged on the floor. If sitting on the floor, experiment with sitting on the edge of a folded blanket or towel to elevate the hips slightly.

3. Check to ensure your head, neck, and back are in alignment. Relax any tension in the jaw or shoulders and rest the hands wherever they feel most comfortable, such as on top of your knees or folded in your lap.

4. Once you feel settled, bring your awareness to your breath. Notice the breath as it flows in and out.

5. As thoughts, sensations, or emotions arise, note the observation by thinking "thought" or "emotion" without judgment, and then bring your focus back to your breath. The goal is not to be a blank slate, but to become more comfortable sitting with your internal experience.

6. When your timer goes off, slowly begin to bring your awareness back to the room by first noticing any sounds or smells and then allowing your eyes to blink open.

7. Take time to observe your surroundings with curiosity before moving on to the next activity in your day.

Non-Judgment

The purpose of any MBSR practice is to step out of the constant cycle of busyness and action to observe your life as it happens. You're not trying to reach any particular state of mind or destination in your healing process; you are being with your experience in the moment and staying present to your life as it unfolds. How many times have you gone on a trip or to a concert and instead of really enjoying yourself in the moment, you got caught up in posting to social media? Or perhaps you didn't apply to a job you really wanted because your inner monologue said you weren't qualified. Judgment can be a saboteur, convincing you that you are not good enough or that what others want is better, all the while missing the truth. This impacts what dreams you do or don't pursue. Unfortunately, the mind can be loud and distracting, like a sports commentator giving you a play-by-play and narrating each experience. You place value judgments on every experience, labeling them as positive or negative.

Through mindfulness, you can begin to take on the role of impartial observer, to notice whatever comes into your awareness—thoughts, emotions, sensations, images, or memories—without judgment. Everything you notice just *is*; nothing is more important or valuable than the rest. Non-judging allows you to step out of the reactivity cycle and into fully living your life.

As you begin to practice the different meditations and mindfulness exercises in this book, you will get to know your judgments very well. You may notice judgments about the practices themselves, whether positive or negative, or you may notice judgments about yourself doing the practices, again positive or negative. That's okay: those assessments will continue to happen, as humans are hardwired with a negativity bias. Identifying the "bad" has historically kept us alive. The purpose of non-judging is not to eliminate judgment altogether, but to become an impartial observer of the process. When you do notice a judgment or critique arise, I invite you to practice noting the judgments just as you would thoughts, being curious about them, and then watching them float away as you would a cloud in the sky.

Mind-Body Awareness

The mind-body connection simply means that what happens in your mind has an impact on the state of your physical health and how your body functions. The experiences happening in your body, such as illness, hunger, or temperature, can have an impact on your emotional state, thoughts, and beliefs. For instance, take a moment to recall the last time you forgot to eat lunch because you got caught up in doing chores at home or were immersed in a work project. How did skipping lunch impact your mood? If you're like most people, you probably felt a bit irritable, or even "hangry" (hungry-angry). Feeling hangry is a common example of the mind-body connection and just how easily your physical state can change your mood.

The mind-body connection goes both ways. Your perceptions, emotions, and thought processes can also greatly influence your physical state. For instance, consider a time when you misinterpreted a conversation with someone. Perhaps you mistakenly thought they disapproved of your work because they were grumpy when they talked to you about it. Their mood, which could have just been a result of them skipping lunch, triggered your feelings of anxiety and fear of rejection. Your perception of the conversation sparked an emotional response, which then ignited a stress reaction in your body. This stress response can throw you into fight-flight-freeze mode, which then causes your immune and digestive systems to shut down. You begin to have indigestion, catch the cold that's been going around the office, or have a chronic condition flare up. This is just one example of how common and powerful the mind-body connection is.

You can nurture this mind-body connection in a positive way through the practice of mindfulness. Instead of unconsciously reaching for coping methods such as comfort eating or losing track of time on social media, you can instead listen to your needs and self-soothe through breathing or self-compassion.

The way to cultivate and strengthen your mind-body connection is through practicing one of the foundational exercises of MBSR: the Body Scan Meditation. As Jon Kabat-Zinn says in his book *Full Catastrophe Living*, the body scan is the foundation for all other meditation practices (2013). You can practice this exercise at any time, although to get the most benefit it is helpful to practice daily for at least two weeks (Kabat-Zinn, 2013).

The goal of the body scan is not to achieve any particular result or state of calm; it is to practice being with yourself in the present moment without judgment. You are building a relationship with your body and becoming more comfortable in stillness. If you find yourself constantly falling asleep during the body scan, you can try practicing with your eyes open. This may indicate a need for more rest or the surfacing of uncomfortable emotions or trauma. If this is the case, it can be helpful to seek the support of a trained psychotherapist or your medical provider.

BODY SCAN MEDITATION

These steps will guide you through a body scan meditation. An audio recording of this meditation is available at AprilSnowConsulting.com/stress-workbook.

1. Set aside at least 30 minutes of uninterrupted time for this exercise.

2. Settle into a comfortable lying-down position. You could choose to be on the floor (on a yoga mat, blanket, or carpet) or in bed. I personally like to have a pillow or bolster under my knees to support my lower back and a blanket to keep me warm. If lying down doesn't feel accessible or you worry about falling asleep, you can sit up instead.

3. Once you feel settled, bring your awareness to your breath. Notice the breath as it flows in through the nostrils and out through the mouth, and feel your belly rise and fall.

4. Allow your awareness to expand outward to your whole body, noticing any thoughts, feelings, or sensations that are present. There's nothing to do or change; just notice yourself in this moment without judgment.

continues »

5. Slowly begin to shift your attention to your left foot, starting at the toes and moving slowly up to the left hip, focusing on one section of the left leg at a time.

6. Imagine your breath is flowing into each part of the body as you bring your full attention there. Notice the presence of any sensations, thoughts, emotions, or imagery as you scan through each part. If there is an absence of feeling or sensation, that is okay, too.

7. Repeat steps 5 and 6 with your right leg.

8. Next, bring your awareness to your pelvis and hips, then to the front and back of the torso. As you move through your belly and heart center, pay close attention to any sensations, thoughts, or emotions that you are aware of.

9. Shift your attention to your left hand, starting at the fingertips, and move slowly up to the left shoulder, focusing on one section of the left arm at a time. Repeat with your right arm.

10. Notice the state of your neck and head, breathing into the front and back of each part.

11. Lastly, bring your attention back to your whole body, all at once. What are you aware of? What, if anything, feels different compared to the start of your practice?

12. Give yourself time to slowly transition out of your practice and back into the rest of your day, or prepare for sleep if you're practicing before bedtime.

Self-Inquiry

Self-inquiry is at the heart of every mindfulness activity, whether formal or informal, and is synonymous with cultivating awareness of your internal experience. Through the practice of self-inquiry, you can reflect inward in order to get to know yourself at a deeper level. Understanding the cycles and connections between your thoughts, emotional reactions, and physical sensations can help you make changes to relieve stress and increase overall well-being.

One example of the importance of self-inquiry is becoming aware of the need to set boundaries in relationships. If you constantly feel exhausted or irritable after you spend time with a particular friend, but it is unclear why, you need to look deeper within. Perhaps this friend is loyal and kind, so until you look more closely, you don't realize that they are actually taking more time than you want to give. After you spend time with this friend, you sit in your car quietly for a few minutes and become aware of how tired you are. You had only intended to go to lunch, but then ended up running errands for a few hours and now won't have time to take care of your own to-do list. There may not be anything wrong with this friendship, it's just that you and your friend have different needs. With a bit of compromise, you can preserve the friendship. This is the power of self-inquiry in action, as part of an informal mindfulness practice.

As you go through each mindfulness exercise or meditation in this book, it can be helpful to observe and record your insights. When you are still and paying attention to your internal landscape, so many ideas and nuggets of self-awareness can surface that have been buried under the noise of your fast-paced life. You may be so disconnected from yourself that you don't even realize how stressed you are until you look within and ask yourself:

▸ How am I?

▸ What do I need in this moment?

▸ Are there obstacles to meeting these needs?

You can use the following log or copy it into a journal to hold your reflections for both informal or formal practices. You can also reflect back on your records to see which practices serve you the most and at what time of day.

Date/Time

Length of Practice

Practice Type/Description

Thoughts, Emotions, Sensations
Prior to Starting Your Practice

Thoughts, Emotions, Sensations
During Your Practice

Thoughts, Emotions, Sensations
After Your Practice

Practice

I can say from personal experience that showing up for mindfulness practice every day is not always easy. Even though I love reflecting inward, have been practicing yoga and meditation for years, and often experience immediate calm and clarity from my practice, I still struggle from time to time. There are so many things calling for my attention and so much pressure to be productive, now more than ever before. Even when I know the research and see the benefits, it can be tempting to stay in bed a little longer in the morning or work a little longer in the evening instead of showing up for myself.

Once you do get into a rhythm with your practice, it becomes easier to overcome the resistance, because the exercises themselves are more familiar and you have experienced the stress-reduction and health benefits firsthand. Think of mindfulness just like any routine, such as brushing your teeth or exercising. It's most helpful when you practice every day. According to researchers at the University of Houston, building a routine is most effective when you make one or two behavioral changes at a time (Arlinghaus & Johnston, 2018). The formal MBSR curriculum slowly adds in meditation practices over eight weeks, maintaining a consistent routine throughout. I would suggest taking a similar approach as you move through this workbook. Instead of speeding through and integrating all the practices at once, try one or two of the meditations per week, practicing every day. For instance, you can start by practicing the Simple Breathing Meditation (page 16) and Body Scan Meditation (page 11) every day for the first week or two before incorporating other exercises. Everyone's experience is unique, and although you may notice a decrease in stress after just a few sessions, studies show the long-term effects and brain changes associated with a mindfulness practice can take up to eight weeks to develop.

Mindfulness truly does become a lifestyle, and like me, you may find yourself naturally bringing mindfulness to everyday moments. The most important part is just showing up to your practice and for yourself each day. The amount of time and the exercises you practice can vary depending on what works for you. I'll offer suggestions for building a daily practice of your own in the next chapter.

MEDITATIONS TO RETURN TO

Consistent practice is the key to easily accessing the stress-reduction and health benefits of mindfulness, but attempting to incorporate a regular practice into your daily schedule can feel overwhelming or impossible. What better way to build your mindfulness muscle than to incorporate mindfulness into activities you already do every day: breathing, walking, and eating?

The following mindfulness exercises offer accessible ways to become more in touch with your moment-to-moment experiences. As you begin connecting to your body and checking in with your emotional state, you can more easily manage stress and accept your needs without judgment.

SIMPLE BREATHING MEDITATION

The breath is your greatest tool to calm anxiety and stress because it's always with you and is simple to use, yet it has a powerful ability to quickly calm your nervous system. Keep this simple breathing exercise in your self-care toolbox for when you're feeling anxious, overwhelmed, or frazzled. An audio recording of this meditation is available at AprilSnowConsulting .com/stress-workbook.

1. Start by closing your eyes or gazing downward.

2. Bring awareness to your breath, noticing its natural rhythm as it flows in and out.

3. Observe the pace and quality of the breath in this moment, without judgment or needing to change anything. Just notice.

4. As you slowly breathe in through the nostrils, say to yourself, "Breath moving in."

5. As you slowly breathe out of the mouth, say to yourself, "Breath moving out."

6. Continue to slowly breathe in and out at your own pace until you feel your body start to relax and unwind. Take as much time as you need for this process to happen.

7. Slowly open your eyes and continue your day.

SIMPLE WALKING MEDITATION

When sitting or breathing meditations aren't accessible or don't invoke a sense of calm, it can be helpful to meet your body in movement. The bilateral stimulation of walking can also be very helpful to process emotions and decrease stress. This simple walking meditation can be practiced inside or outside in a quiet setting. An audio recording of this meditation is available at AprilSnowConsulting.com/stress-workbook.

1. Start by standing with both feet planted firmly on the ground. Hands can rest at your sides or wherever they feel most comfortable.

2. Take a deep breath in through your nostrils, and as you exhale, bring awareness to your left foot and then the right foot.

3. Breathe in, feeling the sensations as you lift your left foot and place your heel on the ground in front of you.

4. Breathe out as you gently press your whole left foot on the ground and allow the weight of your body to rock forward.

5. Breathe in, feeling the sensations as you lift your right foot and place your heel on the ground in front of you.

6. Breathe out as you gently press your whole right foot on the ground and allow the weight of your body to rock forward.

7. Continue to sync your breath with your movement, focusing on the breath and the sensations of your feet touching the ground. If your mind wanders, that's okay: simply redirect your attention back to the process.

8. After a few rounds, step your feet next to each other and take a pause. Without judgment, observe the quality of your thoughts and any physical sensations, and take in your surroundings.

9. Return to walking normally or move on to your next activity.

SIMPLE EATING MEDITATION

Have you ever eaten something so fast or mindlessly that you barely recognized what it tasted like? Food is one of my favorite forms of comfort, but I can often lose myself in the process of eating. This meditation can help you slow down to enjoy the whole eating experience. An audio recording of this meditation is available at AprilSnowConsulting.com/stress-workbook.

1. Arrange a snack or meal in front of you.

2. Sitting quietly and with full attention, pause to notice the colors, textures, and aroma of your food.

3. Using your fingers, feel the textures and temperature.

4. Notice the sensations in your stomach and mouth as you observe the food.

5. Slowly take a bite, experiencing the textures and tastes in your mouth.

6. Bring awareness to how the food's taste and textures change as you mindfully chew.

7. Without hurrying, notice the sensations in your throat and stomach as you swallow this first bite.

8. Take a moment to pause and reflect on what this experience of mindful eating was like for you before transitioning to your next activity.

CHAPTER REFLECTIONS

▶ Mindfulness is simply being aware of the present moment without judgment and can be practiced in any situation throughout the day, such as eating, walking, waiting, or doing chores.

▶ Meditation, on the other hand, is a more formal practice of setting aside time to focus on the breath, physical sensations, thoughts, and emotions.

▶ Self-inquiry can support you as you deepen self-awareness following your informal mindfulness and formal meditation practices.

▶ Although it can be challenging to commit at first, setting aside at least 30 minutes per day to engage in mindfulness has been proven to result in a variety of long-term mental and physical health benefits.

▶ After eight weeks of daily practice, the brain literally begins to rewire, which can produce increased memory and attention, more empathy, less reactivity to stress, better emotional regulation, lower anxiety and stress levels, and fewer ruminating thoughts.

02

Mindfulness in Daily Life

There can be many obstacles to beginning (or returning to) a daily mindfulness routine, but if you wait for your life to be perfect, you'll never start. As you'll learn in this chapter, consistency is important in order to receive the full stress-reduction and health benefits of a mindfulness practice. I'll help you explore what obstacles may create difficulty in carving out time for yourself, as well as how and when to start your practice. This chapter will also explore the importance of letting go of judgmental thinking, how to engage in self-inquiry to establish your internal compass, and the impact of the brain-gut connection on your overall health.

INVITING MINDFULNESS
INTO YOUR DAY

Being a bit of a perfectionist, I began to have this idea that my practice was sacred, and therefore it could only be done in ideal conditions. I imagined waking up with the sunrise to do my yoga and meditation before slowly easing into the rest of my day. As we all know, it's very difficult to maintain that perfectly controlled atmosphere in everyday life. If you wait until you feel 100 percent ready, until the house is fully quiet, until you feel inspired, until your to-do list is empty, you'll never show up to your practice. Over the years I have learned that progress is better than perfection. Showing up on your yoga mat with a toddler or pet joining in or sitting in meditation for a few minutes in the evening after a marathon workday is better than not at all.

I see mindfulness as a relationship that needs to be nurtured regularly to survive and thrive. How do we maintain our relationships? A little bit at a time: a text message during the day to say hello, checking in about your day in the evenings, or a special date night. Translate that concept to mindfulness, and that looks like sitting quietly for a few minutes before lunch to notice your breath, doing a body scan in the evening and journaling about your reflections, or setting aside an hour or two on the weekends to practice yoga and seated meditation. The beauty of a mindfulness practice, especially following the mindfulness-based stress reduction (MBSR) model, is that you have a variety of options that you can customize to fit your lifestyle. If you're a working parent in a relationship, you are going to need a different routine than a single person with a flexible schedule.

There's a line from Jon Kabat-Zinn's book *Full Catastrophe Living* that really woke me up: "You don't have to like it, you just have to do it" (2013). Some days you won't want to sit on your meditation cushion, eat dinner without looking at your phone, or be in the present moment all by yourself without distractions, but you know how much better you feel at the end of the mindfulness process. You know that when you don't practice, your emotional sponge becomes saturated, thoughts pile up unprocessed, and you become disconnected from your physical needs. After some time, you'll begin to notice the difference in yourself when you skip practice: foggy brain, more irritability, difficulty making decisions, less physical comfort, and more stress. It's okay if you can't show up exactly when or how much you want to. The most important part of mindfulness is maintaining that relationship, keeping the familiarity intact so you don't have to reinvent the wheel each time.

The more you practice, even if just for a few minutes, the easier it is to build your mindfulness muscle. Be patient with yourself as you get acquainted with this new part of your routine, as studies show the ability to form a new habit can vary widely. On average, people take 66 days to form a new habit, which lines up with the MBSR eight-week program (Lally et al., 2009). At the end of this chapter, you'll learn how to find space and integrate a mindfulness practice into your life.

MEDITATION: THE FOUNDATION OF MINDFULNESS

Whether you are new to meditation or have been practicing for some time, it can be challenging to find the time or motivation to engage in a formal practice. If you are currently feeling stressed out, which is highly likely considering you picked up this book, it probably feels overwhelming to add one more item to your already overflowing to-do list. How will you find time each and every day? I can completely understand this struggle. Typically, when someone is feeling overextended, self-care practices are the first to go. It's much easier to sacrifice something for yourself rather than letting down the people around you. The truth is that showing up for yourself is not optional: it's necessary to create a sustainable lifestyle over the long run. Luckily, you only need about 10 minutes per day to receive the anxiety- and stress-reducing benefits of meditation (Xu et al., 2017). By carving out 10 minutes to sit quietly and focus on your breath, you can actually create more capacity to tackle your responsibilities and engage with your busy life.

The idea of finding time for yourself to sit quietly and reflect might sometimes sound very inviting. There are times when I feel particularly introspective and can spend hours in my bubble doing yoga, meditating, and journaling. Everyone oscillates between excitement and resistance. Whether you can dedicate 10 minutes or an hour per day, start where you are, because a little goes a long way.

In the MBSR program at the Center for Mindfulness at the University of Massachusetts, participants practice six days per week. When they are forming a new habit, the repetition is most important. Studies show that missing a session doesn't impact the habit formation process as long as consistency is present overall (Lally et al., 2009). Practicing daily helps create an automatic response, so you'll start to show up without much effort after about two months, or sooner for some people (Lally, et al., 2009). Imagine incorporating just 10 minutes of seated meditation into your morning or bedtime routine. After a while, you'll show up on your meditation cushion because it's just part of your routine, like brushing your teeth.

On paper, this may sound simple, but in reality it may feel difficult to know exactly how to get started or when to practice. Generally, meditating in the morning is a great way to set a calm and focused tone for the day, plus all your activities and interactions won't be filling your quiet space. If you are a morning person, have a flexible schedule, or don't have little ones to tend to as soon as you wake up, by all means, practice in the morning. However, if your mornings are too full or you're nocturnal like me, early practice may not align with your natural rhythm or schedule. You can meditate anytime and still receive the benefits. It may just take a bit more time for the sediment to settle, for your body and mind to transition from busy to still. This process can feel uncomfortable at first, as it's hard to be with your thoughts, feelings, and sensations—that's why our lives are often so full of distractions.

The most difficult, but probably the most helpful, time to practice is during or after a stressful event. When I come home after an emotional day of seeing my psychotherapy clients, sometimes I just want to eat some comfort food and watch a movie. What this usually does is distract me from the difficult feelings instead of allowing me to work through them. When I choose to do some stretching on my yoga mat, spend a few minutes checking in with my breath, and journal about what I'm feeling, I can set the stress of my day down instead of allow it to hang out in the background of my mind, waiting for me to go to sleep. Remember that practicing mindfulness helps calm those ruminating thoughts that nag at you after a stressful day. The following meditations will help you get started.

MINDFUL MORNING MEDITATION

Meditation doesn't always have to happen sitting on the cushion. Meet yourself where you are to start your day off mindfully with this simple morning check-in. An audio recording of this meditation is available at AprilSnowConsulting.com/stress-workbook.

1. When you wake up in the morning, take a moment to pause before you look at your phone or hop out of bed to get your coffee.

2. Keeping your eyes closed, notice your body lying on the bed, feeling the support of the bed underneath you and the weight of the blankets around you.

3. Feel your breath moving in and out, feeling your belly rise and fall on each breath.

4. Take a moment to set an intention for the day. How do you want to feel today? What actions will help you feel that way?

5. When you're ready, allow your eyes to slowly adjust to being awake and take in your surroundings before starting your day.

MEDITATION FOR A STRESSFUL DAY

This is a meditation for those days that leave you feeling depleted and over-stimulated. For added benefit, practice this meditation under a weighted blanket, with a heating pad, or while taking an Epsom salt bath. After the meditation, be gentle with yourself for the rest of the evening. Have a cup of herbal tea or get into bed early. An audio recording of this meditation is available at AprilSnowConsulting.com/stress-workbook.

1. Find any comfortable position and bring your eyes to a close or low gaze (looking down into your lap).

2. Without placing any judgment, take a moment to notice the pace and quality of your breath. Is it fast, shallow, or labored? Just be aware of the state of your breath as it moves in and out.

3. Bring awareness to your physical body. Where do you feel tension, heaviness, pain, or numbness? As you breathe in, imagine sending cleansing, nourishing energy to those parts. As you breathe out, imagine softening and releasing whatever you are holding on to in this moment. Continue to breathe, and if it feels right, add a big audible sigh on the exhale.

4. Notice if your body wants to move or stretch in any way, and perhaps roll the neck from side to side, twist the torso, or bring the knees up to the chest and give yourself a hug.

5. Continue breathing and stretching for a few more minutes, then slowly bring your body back to stillness and open your eyes.

LEARNING THE ROLE OF IMPARTIAL OBSERVER

Your mindfulness practice helps you shift out of noisy commentator mode and into the impartial observer role that I spoke of in the previous chapter. Taking the stance of the observer allows you to be more present to your life as it unfolds. You begin to witness instead of critique. Remember that the goal is not to eliminate judgmental thinking altogether, as your brain is wired to assess and scan. The goal is to unhook from this tendency in order to see your experiences more clearly and with less bias.

Judgment is common to all humans: it's a tool we use to understand our complicated world. The problem is that judgments can become absolutes and create limitations. Ever notice that as soon as your inner critic shows up, your confidence melts away? Or you make an assumption about someone and realize later you were completely wrong? I've definitely been there and have almost missed out on important friendships, job opportunities, and feeling confident in myself. It's natural to fill in the details with assumptions when you don't have the whole story, but you want to make sure those assumptions don't become obstacles. Let's look more closely at how judgments can play out in your life.

Comparing yourself with others is so common, especially on social media. When you see someone's "highlight reel" online, miss out on a promotion at work, or have an argument, you may quickly jump to that shame-filled place of "I'm bad" or "I'm not good enough." There is this assumption that you are only valuable if your life is perfect or you're happy all the time, but this is absolutely not true or even attainable. You're just a human doing the best you can with what you have. Mindfulness helps you have more compassion for yourself and let go of the pressure to be perfect.

Another area of your life where judgment plays a starring role is in your interactions with others. Often a detail about someone triggers a feeling in you, causing you to make a judgment about them, either positive or negative. Perhaps their tone of voice reminds you of your loving grandmother and you feel soothed, or their lack of boundaries reminds you of a manipulative ex-partner and you can't get away fast enough. You think you know the whole story, but you are really taking a template in your mind and applying it blindly to this new person. This is why mindfulness is so important: it helps you calm your emotions and detach from your assumptions to see your current reality more clearly.

Self-judgment and judgment of others show up in so many areas. You can judge your thoughts, behaviors, emotions, physical appearance, success, productivity, status—you can even judge how good you are at meditating. Early in college, I had a friend who was very spiritual, and I would often compare myself to her. I judged the beginning of my mindfulness journey as inferior to where she was, years into her practice. This became a big obstacle to finding my own way and led me to instead follow someone else's path. Taking a non-judgmental stance helps you take in the full picture of your own experience instead of comparing it to someone else's. In the process, you can slow down the flood of emotions, soften your inner critic, and lower your stress reactivity.

How can you practice non-judgment in an effort to relieve stress? The simplest way is to observe your thoughts in meditation, such as in the Simple Breathing Meditation (page 16) or Simple Seated Meditation (page 8) from chapter 1. You can also take the observer approach from your meditation practice out into the world. To get an idea of what that might look like, imagine you're at the beach on a crisp autumn day. There's no one there but you, the waves are calm, and the sky is clear with a few clouds. You relax on a blanket with your hands folded behind your head and watch the clouds slowly float by. In this moment, you are quiet as you note the quality and shape of the clouds. There is no critique or comparison, just being present to what you see around you. This is the observer in action, noticing and witnessing without any critique.

Instead of placing a value on your experiences, interactions, or self-worth, the observer just names the facts. In the exercises that follow, you will practice reflecting on your day and social interactions without judgment.

Daily Review Exercise

When you think about your day, your thoughts may be filled with judgments and comparisons. Due to your negativity bias as a human being, your mind can immediately jump to where you came up short or what you didn't like. This exercise will help you take a matter-of-fact approach to reflecting on your day. Make a copy of these questions or write your reflections in a journal.

List what happened throughout your day without judgments or comparisons, focusing only on the facts (behaviors and observations). See the chart of examples for guidance.

Example:

With Judgment	Without Judgment
Woke up later than I wanted to at 9 a.m.	Woke up at 9 a.m.
Only meditated 10 minutes instead of 30	Meditated for 10 minutes
Ate pizza for lunch instead of a salad	Ate pizza for lunch
Didn't say as much as Jeff in the staff meeting	Answered two questions in the staff meeting
Wasted time after work	Watched a movie after work

What thoughts, emotions, or images surfaced as you read through
your daily review?

_____

_____

_____

_____

How does taking a non-judgmental approach shift your perception of
your day?

_____

_____

_____

_____

Try this exercise as part of your evening mindfulness routine; it pairs
perfectly with the Weekly Gratitude Practice (page 152).

Releasing Judgment Toward Others

Although you are probably the most critical of yourself, judging can also interfere with how you perceive others and your ability to build relationships. In this exercise, you will practice setting aside your judgments to see someone as they are, including their strengths and the many layers of their personality. Choose someone who you have consciously judged in the past. It could be a family member, coworker, neighbor, or anyone you have regular contact with.

Describe the person's physical appearance (e.g., height, hair and eye color, style of dress).

_____

_____

_____

Do they work? If so, what do they do and where do they work?

_____

_____

_____

Where do they live? Do they live alone or with family?

_____

_____

_____

Are they single, partnered, or married? Do they have children? If so, how many?

_____

_____

_____

What are some other facts you know about them (e.g., birthplace, age, interests/hobbies)?

_____

_____

_____

_____

What do you have in common with this person? List as many commonalities as you can, such as workplace, age, gender, hair color, hometown, interests, etc.

_____

_____

_____

_____

Take a moment to look over your observations of this person as a human, separate from your perceptions of them. What thoughts, emotions, or sensations arise?

_____

_____

_____

_____

_____

After completing this exercise, notice if your interactions with this person or ability to connect with them have changed.

THE KEY TO WELL-BEING

In the previous chapter, you learned about the power of the mind-body connection and the part it plays in your physical and mental health. Being aware of this interplay between your physical, mental, and emotional realms can have a significant impact on your life. Your body holds a lot of wisdom and often gives you clues about your needs and emotional experiences. Think of a time when you had butterflies in your stomach from anxiety, heartburn after a stressful day, or a gut feeling about someone you just met for the first time. Even looking at the phrases we use to describe these common manifestations of emotional experience is telling. According to the American Psychological Association, research is showing more and more proof that the gut can influence "emotional behavior, pain perception and how the stress system responds" (Carpenter, 2012). This brain-gut connection goes two ways, as the brain can also impact gut health. For instance, even mild stress levels can cause digestive health issues and decrease immune functioning (Carpenter, 2012).

There is a clear mind-body connection that you can tap into to learn more about yourself and your needs in any given moment. When I am stressed, I unconsciously hunch my shoulders or tense my feet. When I find myself in these postures, I know it's time to slow down, take a few breaths, and check in with myself.

Paying attention to your body, thoughts, and emotional landscape can feel overwhelming or scary, especially if you have been focusing outward or have experienced trauma in the past. There are many reasons you may become uncomfortable looking within yourself and connecting to your body. Perhaps you're struggling to meet the expectations of society to look a certain way, or have had some type of physical or emotional trauma. For the first 18 years of my life, I learned to disavow my emotions because my feelings were overwhelming. It wasn't until I had the opportunity to heal through psychotherapy and my mindfulness practice that I began to reunite with myself. I discovered a deep well of intuition and guidance that I'd never had access to before. Be patient with yourself, and give yourself time for your frozen awareness to thaw.

The Body Scan Meditation (page 11) is the foundation of getting reacquainted with your thoughts, feelings, and physical sensations, but there are many opportunities to check in with yourself every day. The next two exercises will help you bring mind-body awareness to ordinary activities, such as taking a shower or preparing a meal. Feel free to apply this same conscious mindset to any activity throughout your day.

Listening to Your Body's Wisdom

Take a few moments to reflect on some of the ways your body expresses emotions or gives you clues about your needs. Include both positive and negative experiences. For each area listed, write down sensations you commonly feel. If nothing, you can write down neutral or numb.

Head _____

Example: Aching or clear

Throat _____

Example: Tight or sore

Shoulders _____

Example: Tense or painful

Torso _____

Example: Chest tight or belly soft

Arms _____

Example: Stiff or tingling

Pelvis _____

Example: Tight or loose

Legs _____

Example: Achy or restless

Whole Body _____

Example: Heavy or numb

When your body is experiencing these feelings, what is it trying to tell you?

Example: When I feel lightness in my whole body, I know I am well-rested.
Example: When I get chronic headaches, I know I am overstimulated or overworked.
Example: When my belly feels soft, I know I feel safe with someone.

Example: When I get tense talking to someone, I know I need to set a boundary.

We each have unique experiences with the ways our bodies talk to us and how our emotions show up in physical form, if at all. How does it feel to focus on the relationship between your mind and body?

Mindful Shower

The shower is often the one space completely without distractions. It's where you process your day, imagine past and future conversations, and come up with your best ideas. If possible, try this exercise before bed.

1. Take a moment to gather anything you'll need after your shower, such as a towel, pajamas, or moisturizer.

2. Before you turn on the water, take a moment to check in with yourself.

    a) How am I feeling in this moment?
    b) What is my stress level before getting into the shower: low, moderate, or high?

3. Notice the sound and temperature of the water as you turn it on. Really tune in to this delightful sensory experience, as if you are a child taking your first shower.

4. As you shower, bring to mind what was stressful about your day and imagine the water washing those stressors down the drain, creating a sense of lightness within and around your body.

5. When you're ready, turn off the shower and notice the sounds of the water fading away into silence.

6. Feel the texture and temperature of your towel as you dry off, then feel the clothes on your freshly washed skin.

7. Before leaving the bathroom, take a moment to check in with yourself.

    a) How am I feeling in this moment?
    b) What is my stress level post-shower: low, moderate, or high?

Experiment with approaching your showers mindfully a few times each week, noticing the difference in your stress levels and ability to be present.

Mindful Cooking

Applying your mindfulness practice to cooking is a great opportunity to slow down and engage the senses. For this exercise, prepare a simple meal, such as oatmeal or soup.

1. Start by noticing your feet planted firmly on the ground of your kitchen floor.

2.   Bring your awareness to your belly, feeling it rise as your breath moves in and fall as you exhale. How hungry do you feel in this moment?

3.   Hear the hiss of the fire beneath the pan or the sizzle of the food cooking.

4.   Smell the aromas moving from the pan toward your nose. What does it smell like? What does it remind you of?

5.   Feel the metal of the pan's handle in one hand and the texture of the spoon in the other. How does the texture and temperature feel on your skin?

6.   See the ingredients in the pan slowly transforming as they cook, as you gently stir with your spoon. Perhaps notice the steam slowly rising up and feel the warmth on your face.

7.   Notice your experience of waiting for the food to cook. Are you salivating? Do you feel excited or impatient for the food to be ready?

Mindfulness is simply noticing what's present for us in each moment, without judgment or the need to change anything. Now, make note of what came up for you during this cooking exercise.

Thoughts:

Feelings:

Physical sensations:

_____

_____

Images or memories:

_____

_____

What felt difficult?

_____

_____

_____

_____

What felt enjoyable?

_____

_____

_____

_____

Since you may cook frequently, this is a great opportunity to incorporate mindful awareness. Start with cooking one mindful meal per week and build up from there.

CREATING A RELATIONSHIP WITH YOURSELF

Self-inquiry is a process of exploring your inner world, reflecting on your experiences, and processing your emotions. I like to think of it as creating a relationship with yourself—mind, body, and spirit. I personally believe a combination of lengthy conversations and brief check-ins is the best approach to getting to know yourself more deeply, and I have included different options throughout this chapter.

Some of the benefits of practicing self-inquiry and being more self-aware include:

▸ Living in accordance with your personal values

▸ Understanding your needs

▸ Setting the right goals for yourself

▸ Knowing when you need to set limits

▸ Creating more awareness of your thoughts, emotions, and sensations

▸ Processing your experiences

▸ Reducing stress levels

▸ Deepening self-compassion and emotional regulation

▸ Listening to your intuition and inner wisdom

Think about any other benefits of self-inquiry you have experienced in the past or hope to tap into going forward. Would you add anything to this list?

How do you cultivate self-inquiry in your daily life? Modern life has made it increasingly difficult to get quiet and listen to the subtle voice within. Because of this, the most effective way to nourish your self-inquiry practice is to schedule time for yourself. If you have already incorporated meditation into your routine, you can include your self-inquiry practice then. If not, set aside time during some part of your day to get quiet and engage in the practices listed here. Choose an item from your to-do list that you could delegate or delete, and think about how you can commit to making this time for yourself. Personally, I engage in structured self-inquiry before bed by journaling about my day. I allow whatever comes to mind to flow onto the page without judgment. This allows me to reflect on my day in a structured way and notice what emotions have surfaced as a result. It can also be helpful to journal in the morning, allowing you to process and clear away material from your dreams, worries about your day, or other thoughts.

What types of self-inquiry call to you?

JOURNALING: Write down your thoughts and feelings.

DAYDREAMING: Allow your imagination to wander.

WRITING: Channel your experiences into a story or draft a letter to yourself.

SEATED MEDITATION: Sit quietly with your thoughts, emotions, and physical sensations.

ART: Make a collage or create a vision board.

MOVEMENT: Connect with yourself through dance, walking, or yoga.

TAROT CARDS: Use the cards as a guide.

PSYCHOTHERAPY: Enlist the help of an impartial other.

SELF-TALK: Have a verbal dialogue with yourself.

Self-inquiry will occur naturally during your mindfulness practices but can be deepened with more intentional self-reflection. The next two exercises will help you start to engage in self-inquiry throughout your day. Experiment with different practices to see what helps you get more in touch with your thoughts and feelings.

Self-Reflective Journaling

Journaling is a helpful tool for processing your experiences. You can try either structured or unstructured journaling, depending on what feels right for you. I recommend experimenting with both styles, setting aside 5 to 10 minutes first thing in the morning or right before you go to sleep. You can begin in the spaces provided or use a separate journal, finding the time that works best for you.

Option One: Unstructured Journaling

You can journal in a stream-of-consciousness style, also known as a "brain dump," where you simply write down whatever thoughts, memories, feelings, or images come to mind. Don't worry about sentence structure or grammar, just put words and/or drawings onto paper. You can engage in a dialogue with yourself, write about not knowing what to write—anything goes as long as you leave judgment aside! This method can be very freeing, as it takes away the pressure to be perfect.

Option Two: Structured Journaling

If you are new to journaling, unsure what to write about, or feeling stuck, it can help to start with specific prompts. Use these questions to spark your self-reflective writing.

- What thoughts, feelings, and sensations am I aware of in this moment?

- What am I grateful for?

- What was difficult about today?

Once you complete your journaling, you may want to spend a few moments looking over what you just wrote or noticing how you feel.

Replacing Social Media with Self-Inquiry

There are many opportunities for self-inquiry throughout the day that you may miss when looking at your phone, checking email, or scrolling through social media. It's common to lose track of time during these activities. The next time you have the urge to reach for your phone, I invite you to pause and practice these steps. An audio recording of this exercise is available at AprilSnowConsulting.com/stress-workbook.

1. Notice the urge to fill this space with distraction. Where is that coming from?

2. Close your eyes and press your feet firmly into the floor. Feel your feet making contact with the ground and note any sensations in your body.

3. Take a few deep breaths, in through the nose and out through the mouth, pursing your lips as if you were blowing out a candle.

4. Ask yourself, "How am I doing in this moment?" and "What do I need?"

5. What thoughts, emotions, or physical sensations are you aware of? Remember to name your experience without judgment, as if you were narrating a scene in a movie.

6. Take a few more deep breaths.

7. How did it feel to pause and check in with yourself?

This exercise can help you replace the urge for digital distraction with a mindful check-in. When in a rush, simply take a few deep breaths instead of picking up your phone.

BUILDING YOUR MINDFULNESS MUSCLE

Throughout chapters 1 and 2, you've learned about a variety of benefits to your physical and mental health from practicing mindfulness. Perhaps you're excited to experience the benefits for the first time or to reconnect with your practice if you're a seasoned meditator. If you're starting to feel a bit overwhelmed about starting the process or doubtful about finding the time, you are not alone! It's hard to embark upon something new, especially when you're feeling stressed and anxious or are experiencing chronic pain or health struggles. You don't have to feel ready or get it exactly right. The goal is progress, not perfection. Just show up a little every day in order to build your mindfulness muscle.

You wouldn't expect an athlete who skips practices or training sessions to perform their best during a game. More likely, they would lag behind and be out of sync with their teammates. Think of mindfulness as practice and your life as the game. Although we don't always want to show up, practice prepares us to handle the pressure and stress of our lives.

Remember that it's less important *how* you practice mindfulness compared to *how much* you show up. It's okay to build slowly and be imperfect. If you miss a day or have less time to practice, don't let that stop you. The first step in creating your mindfulness routine is thinking about how much time you plan to dedicate to your practice. Do you have time to dedicate 15 to 20 minutes per day? Excellent! Do you have closer to five minutes? That's great, too: Start there. Whatever time you find to dedicate to your mindfulness routine, you will have to prioritize your needs and create space for your own well-being. For some, this practice of self-care might feel edgy or guilt-inducing. It may be hard to say no to others, set boundaries around your time, or ask for help so you can take care of yourself. Brainstorm a few ways you can get your needs met, such as asking for help with childcare, reducing commitments at work, or being less available by phone in the evenings for friends.

Now that we've explored the *how much*, let's talk a bit more about the *how*. There are many options for practicing mindfulness—more than I can explore in this book. If we zoom in from an MBSR perspective, the formal practices include seated meditation, body scan, breath awareness, yoga, and walking, which can be alternated throughout the week once you have established a rhythm to your practice. The informal practice options, such as taking a mindful shower or cooking mindfully, are vast. The more you practice, the more automatic the process will feel.

To start building the foundation of your mindfulness routine, I would suggest focusing on one formal and one informal practice each week, engaging in both every day. I will guide you in choosing your practices in the exercises that follow.

Finding Time for Mindfulness

Set aside time to look at your current schedule. Add a checkmark to this chart for all the times you could make available for your mindfulness practice. It's okay if your availability is limited; the most important thing is to establish a routine of practicing at the same time throughout the week.

	SUN	MON	TUE	WED	THUR	FRI	SAT
5:00 a.m.							
6:00 a.m.							
7:00 a.m.							
8:00 a.m.							
9:00 a.m.							
10:00 a.m.							
11:00 a.m.							
12:00 p.m.							
1:00 p.m.							
2:00 p.m.							

	SUN	MON	TUE	WED	THUR	FRI	SAT
3:00 p.m.							
4:00 p.m.							
5:00 p.m.							
6:00 p.m.							
7:00 p.m.							
8:00 p.m.							
9:00 p.m.							
10:00 p.m.							
11:00 p.m.							

What time(s) could you set aside every day to create a familiar routine? List them below or circle them on the chart.

With your current commitments, how much time could you practice at this time each day? 10 minutes? 30 minutes? 60 minutes?

Are there any changes you need to make to your current schedule or commitments to carve out more time for yourself? If so, what are they?

_____

_____

_____

If you implemented these changes, how much time could you practice at this time each day? 10 minutes? 30 minutes? 60 minutes?

_____

What thoughts, emotions, or physical sensations come up as you imagine making these changes to prioritize your needs?

_____

_____

_____

Give yourself time to implement your new mindfulness schedule and allow for imperfection as you transition into this new routine. It will take time to shift your commitments and dedicate more time to your practice.

Deciding What to Practice

Now that you've carved out time to practice each day (or most days) and figured out how much time you can dedicate to your practice, it's time to identify what meditations or exercises you want to start with.

Formal Meditations	Informal Mindfulness
Seated	**Any activity you bring awareness to, such as:**
Simple Seated Meditation (page 8)	Washing the dishes
Body Scan Meditation (page 11)	Eating a meal
Simple Breathing Meditation (page 16)	Folding laundry
Movement	Taking a shower
Yoga for a Stressful Day (page 124)	Going for a hike
Simple Walking Meditation (page 17)	Walking the dog

Formal Practice

From the menu of options, choose one formal meditation practice you would prefer to focus on over the next one to two weeks. You can find meditation scripts for each formal practice in chapter 1 of this book and a yoga sequence on page 124.

Informal Practice

What are some daily activities that you could bring mindful awareness to?

For the next week, choose one of the activities you listed to focus on each day. If you would like a bit of support getting started, you can start with Mindful Shower (page 36) or Mindful Cooking (page 37) from earlier in this chapter.

I have included a sample schedule for the first three weeks of practice. Feel free to follow this routine or create your own in the empty chart that follows.

Week One Sample

Type	Practice	Length	Schedule
Formal	Simple Breathing Meditation	5 minutes	Mornings at 8 a.m.
Informal	Mindful Shower	10 minutes	Before bed at 9 p.m.

Week Two Sample

Type	Practice	Length	Schedule
Formal	Simple Seated Meditation	10 minutes	Mornings at 8 a.m.
Informal	Mindful Cooking	20 minutes	Dinner at 6 p.m.

Week Three Sample

Type	Practice	Length	Schedule
Formal	Body Scan Meditation	30 minutes	Mornings at 8 a.m.
Informal	Washing the Dishes	10 minutes	After dinner at 7 p.m.

Week One			
Type	**Practice**	**Length**	**Schedule**
Formal			
Informal			

Week Two			
Type	**Practice**	**Length**	**Schedule**
Formal			
Informal			

Week Three			
Type	**Practice**	**Length**	**Schedule**
Formal			
Informal			

You'll notice in the sample schedule that I slowly increased the total amount of combined practice time from 15 minutes the first week to 30 minutes the second week to 40 minutes the third week. It can be helpful to slowly ease into this practice to give yourself time to acclimate to a new routine.

CHAPTER REFLECTIONS

▸ Mindfulness is a relationship that must be nurtured consistently in order to produce the full benefits. The goal is not to be perfect but to show up a little each day until the practice becomes a new habit.

▸ An MBSR-inspired mindfulness practice engages you in present-moment awareness in order to become an impartial observer and build judgment-free relationships with yourself and others.

▸ There is a proven mind-body connection. Practicing mindfulness will awaken you to the messages your body is sending about your stress levels, emotional well-being, and overall health.

▸ The process of self-inquiry during meditation, or through journaling or other practices, helps ensure you're acting in alignment with your values, getting your needs met, and tapping into your intuition.

▸ Studies show that we can receive the stress- and anxiety-reduction benefits of mindfulness by practicing for as little as 10 minutes per day.

03

Mindfulness in Relationships

Think of all the people you come into contact with throughout a typical week, from strangers to close family and friends. There are so many types of relationships to navigate in daily life, each with its own complexities, but you aren't given a relationship manual or any tools to understand how to manage these interactions. Mindfulness can help you get clear on your own needs in relationships, regulate emotions during conflict, and have the clarity to communicate with more ease. In this chapter, you'll learn how to integrate the benefits of meditation into your relationships with others, let go of judgment to listen mindfully, use mind-body awareness to deescalate conflicts, and create deeper connections with loved ones.

THE MINDFUL RELATIONSHIP

You navigate relationships with family, friends, coworkers, partners, spouses, and neighbors every day, but did anyone ever teach you how to clearly communicate in those relationships? Most likely not. Instead, you learned by observing those around you and internalizing the patterns you saw played out in your immediate family. This isn't always the best system, especially if your role models didn't know how to communicate clearly or self-soothe when conflict arose. Thankfully, mindfulness can help you navigate the complexity of being in contact with another person.

Let's face it: relationships of all kinds take work and practice to run smoothly. The uncertainty of relationships can create a lot of stress in your life, but why? From a very primal framework, humans need others to survive, since we spend so much time maturing compared to other species. As a result, research has found that the human brain has evolved to respond to social disconnection and physical pain in similar ways (Eisenberger & Lieberman, 2004). Your body has cleverly utilized the pain response because it's difficult to ignore and therefore forces you to seek connection (Eisenberger & Lieberman, 2004).

Although you have many types of relationships in your life, the most stressful are typically with the people you spend the most time with or the people who are most important to you. This could be your close family members, best friend, or a partner or spouse. Communication issues, especially around getting your needs heard and met, are at the heart of most relationship stress. With a partner or spouse, communication breakdowns often happen around the subjects of housework, money, sex, and parenting, or any area where the division of labor may become unequal. When communication and connection are absent, resentment increases and shared experiences start to evaporate. What's left is a relationship that's all work and no play.

For a relationship to run smoothly, there must be enough space within yourself to notice and hear the other person: to listen and have empathy when they are having a hard day at work, to notice when they throw out a bid for connection such as mentioning a movie they're interested in, or to have the bandwidth to work through a disagreement calmly. According to renowned couples researcher Dr. John Gottman, members of couples who stay together answer their partner's bids for connection 86 percent of the time, whereas members of divorced couples only answer their partner's bids 33 percent of the time (Brittle, 2015). Being attentive in your relationships is necessary for their survival.

This is where mindfulness comes in! As you learned in chapter 1, mindfulness helps you wring out your emotional sponge and calm your own nervous system so you can be more present to your partner, spouse, child, or anyone you are in a relationship with. Imagine two scenarios:

1. You have meetings all day, work through lunch, and then rush home to either immediately start making dinner for your family or go out to meet up with a friend.

2. You work all day, but take a lunch, and meditate for 10 minutes in the car before going into the house to make dinner or to meet up with your friend.

In which scenario will you have more bandwidth to engage with another person? Clearly, in the second scenario you have taken time to slow down and de-stress, creating a bit more capacity to engage with others, manage your emotions, and have the awareness to set boundaries if you need to. In the first scenario, you're probably feeling overstimulated from being *on* all day and are more likely to be irritable, and you may say something out of anger that you later regret.

A University of North Carolina study showed that couples practicing mindfulness displayed decreased stress overall and improved relationship happiness (Carson et al., 2004). Incorporating mindfulness into your daily life not only helps you stay more present to your internal experience and needs, it also helps you manage the stress of relationships.

STRENGTHENING YOUR RELATIONSHIPS USING MEDITATION

Meditation is an introspective and very personal process, so you may be wondering how it can integrate into your relationships. You may also worry that meditation won't benefit your relationship unless your partner or family member practices with you. These are valid questions, as often our most replenishing self-care practices are not shared by the people in our lives. Whether you practice on your own or with a partner, friend, or family member, meditation can have benefits not just for you but for anyone you interact with. That includes your family, friends, coworkers, partner, spouse, children, and neighbors.

As you've learned in previous sections of this book, practicing mindfulness-based stress reduction (MBSR) on a regular basis greatly improves your ability to be aware of your needs, soothe your emotional reactions when you get triggered by people or events, and calm the fight-flight-freeze response when you feel stressed. These benefits allow you to be more available for connection and more clearly communicate your experience without getting caught in the storm of shame and blame that often accompanies conflict.

If you're spending most of your day engaged with other people or in a caregiving role, it's easy to feel depleted. When you start to feel exhausted, you get resentful of others, which leads to irritability and poor communication. Think about how you talk to your partner or family following a long day at work or after sightseeing on vacation. Most likely you don't have much bandwidth to listen, and you may respond in a way that you regret later. This happened when my grandmother was visiting me in California a few years back. After several days in a row of not being able to do my yoga and meditation practice, I was running on empty. At the end of a long day, I found myself feeling overstimulated and irritable toward my grandmother, which is the opposite of how I wanted to engage with her. After reflecting on the moment, which I still remember so clearly, I realized how important my mindfulness practice is to my relationships. Think of your meditation practice as the fuel that gives you the energy to connect and communicate clearly with all the people in your life. Taking time to be aware of your own needs is essential to successfully maintaining your relationships.

If finding the time and space to practice by yourself is proving difficult, you may need to set boundaries around your practice time so other responsibilities do not interfere, or enlist a meditation buddy such as your spouse or a friend to help keep you accountable. Be sure to turn off your phone, let others know you won't be available during that time, and consider asking others for help if you have caregiver responsibilities that need tending to while you're meditating. If your partner or spouse is not practicing with you, perhaps you could ask them for help in getting some quiet time alone.

Whether practiced alone or with others, meditation can help strengthen your relationship connections and communication. If you find yourself feeling depleted by too much connection, you can practice the following Energizing Meditation. If you have someone to meditate with, you can experiment with different types of meditation and then share your experiences in the Creating Connection through Meditation exercise (page 60).

ENERGIZING MEDITATION

Staying engaged and connected with others is rewarding and important for survival, but it can be exhausting and leave you feeling disconnected from yourself, especially if you're an introvert. Keep this simple meditation in your back pocket to refuel your social energy during and after social engagements—step outside briefly if you need to. An audio recording of this meditation is available at AprilSnowConsulting.com/stress-workbook.

1. Close your eyes and take a few slow, deep breaths.

2. As you inhale, imagine your body filling with fresh energy.

3. As you exhale, visualize any problems or emotions that you heard from the other person being cleansed away.

4. Repeat this meditation a few times until you feel calmer and more centered.

5. Slowly open your eyes.

CREATING CONNECTION THROUGH MEDITATION

There are many ways to incorporate meditation into your relationships if you have a receptive partner, friend, or family member. Have a silent meal together and practice the Simple Eating Meditation (page 18), engage in moving meditation by going on a mindful walk or doing yoga together, practice seated meditation in the mornings before breakfast, or do the Body Scan Meditation (page 11) at the end of the day.

After you practice together, spend a few moments sharing your experience. You can take turns listening and reflecting on the following questions:

1. What sensations, thoughts, and emotions were present for you during the practice?

2. How do you feel as a result of the practice?

3. What was meaningful about sharing this practice together?

To ensure each person feels heard and has space to share, take turns playing the role of listener and speaker. The speaker shares as the listener reflects back a brief summary of what they heard in their own words. It's important to hold off on asking questions until the other person has finished speaking. Switch roles, then have space for an open discussion at the end. Thank each other for practicing together.

ACCEPTING OTHERS AS THEY ARE

Your judgments, biases, and assumptions may get in the way of seeing others clearly for who they are, because you may be interpreting their behaviors through the lens of your own experiences. When you interact with another person, you may see a reflection of others who have caused you pain, joy, or other emotions. This is why it's important to step outside of judgment to learn more about an individual's unique experience, needs, and feelings. Assumptions make it easy to lose touch with the present moment and how you may be affecting the relationship, perhaps triggering certain behaviors in the other person. This can create a spiral of miscommunication and conflict.

Playing the role of impartial observer allows you to detach from assumptions, unreasonable expectations, and emotional reactivity. Instead of comparing yourself to another or competing with them, you can tend to your own emotions, communicate your needs clearly, and react with empathy. Instead of making assumptions or judgments, you can instead ask: What story do I have about this person? Have I asked for clarification about my assumptions? What could this person be feeling and needing in this moment? You can also use your self-inquiry skills to check in with yourself and ask: What am I feeling and needing? How could I clearly communicate that in a non-defensive and direct way?

Another important component of this non-judgmental stance is staying in the present moment with the other person. You may judge someone, especially partners, spouses, or anyone who you've had a long history with, based on their past actions or how they've responded to you. By assuming you know how someone will respond or why they are saying or doing something, you lose sight of what's actually happening and create the perfect opportunity for misunderstanding and conflict. Instead, you can approach the interaction with open arms. For instance, if your friend is late to a lunch date with you and they've ignored responsibilities in the past, you may assume that they don't respect your time. However, perhaps this time they got an upsetting phone call before they were about to leave the house or got stuck in traffic. As you're waiting, take a step back to notice what feelings are coming up for you and what story you're building up in your head. Then, give your friend a chance to tell you what actually happened. If a difficult situation made them late, you will feel better having approached them with empathy and understanding. If they did just disrespect your time, then you can share the feelings you noticed.

Another judgment that often surfaces in relationships is comparison. You may assume you're not good enough, smart enough, or successful enough because your life doesn't resemble someone else's. This can create a scenario where you have unreasonable expectations of yourself and don't take into account the full picture of your strengths and achievements. For instance, I had to work to put myself through college and often compared myself to the students who were financially supported by their parents. Looking back, I realize that our situations were very different and each had their own benefits and challenges. Working through school gave me a sense of accomplishment, allowed me to develop skills I still use today, and created many impactful relationships with coworkers. But at the time, comparing my situation to others' blinded me to these benefits.

Taking a stance of self-compassion can buffer you from the negative effects of judgment and social comparison (Choi et al., 2014). Let's explore a few exercises for beginning to practice non-judgment in your relationships with others and yourself.

Mindful Listening

When you are having a conversation with another person, are you concentrating fully on what they're saying, or are you thinking about what to say in response? Often when people are conversing they aren't fully present, focusing instead on opinions or feelings about what the other person is saying. This leaves room for miscommunication and conflict, but being mindfully present to the conversation can create connection.

1. Set the intention to give this person your full, undivided attention for the next few minutes. Clear away any distractions such as your phone, television, or computer.

2. Before getting started, settle into your seat and take a few deep breaths to calm your nervous system and clear your mind.

3. If it helps, you can continue to focus on your breathing throughout the conversation as an anchor to help you stay focused.

4. Instead of making assumptions or filling in the blanks while listening, if something is unclear, ask the speaker for more detail. You can simply say, "Tell me more."

5. Notice if your mind begins to wander to what you want to say in response or judgments begin to arise. Simply note your internal response and bring your awareness back to the speaker.

6. Once the speaker is finished sharing, take a few moments to reflect back what you just heard and ask, "Did I get that right?" Refrain from sharing any opinions or comparisons.

7. Allow the speaker to clarify and share any final thoughts.

8. Once the speaker feels understood, switch roles so you have an opportunity to be the speaker.

Try this exercise once per week with your partner, spouse, best friend, or family member to improve communication.

Mindful Self-Acceptance

As you observe and interact with others around you or scroll through social media, sometimes your inner critic says you don't measure up. It's exhausting and may impact your ability to show up fully in your relationships. Instead, let's practice taking a non-judgmental approach to observing yourself in connection to others. You can practice this while scrolling through your friends' social media accounts, listening to the successes of your coworkers, or participating in any interaction where you feel the urge to compare and judge yourself in relation to another person.

What are the details of this interaction? Name the facts such as the person involved, location, activity, and so forth.

As you listen to the story or observe the update, what do you notice stirring within yourself? Write down any thoughts, feelings, physical sensations, memories, or images that come to your mind.

_____

_____

_____

_____

Bring awareness to any judgments that want to surface, name them as such, and let them float by like a cloud in the sky.

On a scale of 1 to 10, how hard was it to observe without judgment?

1	2	3	4	5	6	7	8	9	10

Easy   Neutral   Difficult

Continue to practice playing the part of the impartial observer as you engage with the people in your life and note how you rate the difficulty of this practice over time.

IMPROVING RELATIONSHIPS USING MIND-BODY AWARENESS

Have you ever gotten caught up in an argument where you lashed out verbally in anger, needed to escape the room quickly, or even felt frozen and couldn't speak? That's because your body was in a state of stress and turned on the fight-flight-freeze response. Although you weren't necessarily in physical danger, underlying fears surfaced, like losing a spouse to divorce, becoming estranged from a trusted support person, or getting fired from a job that you rely on.

All of your relationships are important to you emotionally and for various aspects of your survival, so when a conflict arises, your body responds. Next time you begin to get upset, take note of your body's reaction: you may notice physical signs that your body is preparing for a threat, such as an elevated heart rate, shallow breath, or an upset stomach. When you are in this dysregulated state, you become unable to manage your emotions or think clearly. These physical indicators can help you understand that you've been triggered by someone's actions or words.

When you are mindful of your body's signals, you can intervene early to stop the escalation of conflict. Next, I'll share an example of using mindfulness to work through a conflict in real time.

Imagine you are in the middle of a disagreement with your partner or best friend, who is agitated and upset that you worked late again and missed a special event. Typically, you get swept into the argument and become defensive about working late, but lately you have been trying new mindfulness practices to help you manage your emotions.

As you pause to check in with yourself, you notice your heart rate starting to increase and your breath becoming shallower. At this point, you have two choices. You can continue to get deeper into the argument, reacting from your primitive brain and probably saying something that you will regret later, or you can engage mindfully to step out of the storm that is brewing within. As your loved one is talking, you focus on slowing your breath and orient yourself to a soothing object in the room, noticing its colors and shape.

As you begin to anchor your attention in the present moment, your heart rate starts to slow down a bit and you are able to take a deeper breath, engaging the parasympathetic nervous system. You hear more clearly what your loved one is saying and can access empathy for their frustration. You realize you would also feel upset if they had missed an important event.

Mindfulness not only helps us understand our body's messages, but it also helps us regulate our emotions during difficult conversations. Another helpful component of our mind-body awareness practice is listening to the cues that tell us our needs aren't being met. For instance, if you constantly feel tired or irritable after spending time with someone, you may need to set firmer boundaries with that person or limit the amount of emotional space you're willing to hold for them. If you feel relaxed, excited, or inspired when you are with a friend, then you know this is someone you may feel comfortable spending more time with.

In the exercise that follows, you'll begin to cultivate more mind-body awareness in your relationships and learn how often to engage and mindfully navigate conflict.

Increasing Mind-Body Awareness in Relationships

When spending time with another person, it's easy to lose connection with your own body and emotional state. You get drawn into what they're saying and want to be supportive, but then end up losing track of your own needs and experience. In this exercise, you will practice maintaining self-awareness while simultaneously being in contact with another person.

1.   Notice your body language as you talk to someone. Are you leaning in toward them? Sitting very close?

2.   Take a moment to lean backward or pivot slightly away to create a bit more personal space. How does that feel? Do you need more or less space in this moment?

3.   Bring your awareness to your breath. Is your breath shallow or are you breathing normally? What might that tell you?

4.   Notice how fast your heart is beating. If your heart rate is elevated, what does that tell you?

5.   As you engage in conversation, make a conscious effort to check in with yourself from time to time by asking: How am I feeling in this moment? What is the quality of my thoughts?

6.   If you're feeling engaged and calm, continue the conversation.

7.   If you're feeling distracted or tense, or experiencing shallow breathing or an elevated heart rate, you know this interaction has become stressful or you're out of fuel. Take a moment to step away and take a few deep breaths or end the conversation if you can.

8.   How did it feel to check in and take care of your own needs while interacting with someone else? You may notice that it's easier or more difficult with some people than others.

Navigating Conflicts Mindfully

Conflicts and miscommunications are inevitable in relationships, and when managed properly, they can often help strengthen a connection. When navigating conflict with a significant other or your immediate family, create a game plan ahead of time, when you are clearheaded. Here are a few suggestions to get you started.

What are some signs that you are dysregulated or entering fight-flight-freeze mode? Be specific: elevated tone of voice, phrases you typically use, physical sensations such as a flushed face or shallow breath, or feelings you're aware of such as fear or anger. Ask the other person what they observe, as you may not be aware of everything.

How can you respond when you notice you have become dysregulated? Check all that apply and then add your own ideas.

- [ ] Take a few deep breaths until you begin to feel calm.

- [ ] Orient to the space by finding a soothing object; describe its characteristics.

- [ ] Ask to take a pause for 15 minutes to allow your nervous system to calm down.

What can the other person do to support you?

_____

_____

_____

_____

_____

_____

_____

Next time you find yourself in a conflict, practice your mindfulness skills to notice when you're getting dysregulated and remind the other person what support you need. This may feel clunky or messy at first because it's new, but it will become easier over time.

UNDERSTANDING YOUR NEEDS IN RELATIONSHIPS

Have you ever wished the people in your life could read your mind and know exactly what you need? That would prevent so much conflict and miscommunication, but it's just not possible. For communication to be effective, you first have to know your own needs, and then find ways to express those needs to the person you're talking to. Over time, the people closest to you may notice that when you're quiet it means you're tired, or when you're irritable it means you're hungry, but this level of knowing takes time and isn't foolproof. Self-inquiry, as a part of your mindfulness work, is the path to understanding yourself more deeply and asking, "How am I, who am I, what do I need, do I have the capacity to give, and if so, how much?" This process of introspection helps you identify not only what your needs are but also your boundaries, which are necessary to sustain any relationship long-term.

The practice of self-inquiry can be formal or informal and can include seated meditation, journaling, creating art, talking to a therapist, or any practice for exploring your inner world. It always involves checking on your internal experience, including the quality and content of your thoughts, the layers of your emotional landscape, and the sensations your body is feeling, as well as memories, imagery, dreams, and so on. Self-inquiry is about developing a deep relationship with yourself first. When you understand your emotional reactions, thought processes, and physical sensations, including how and why they show up, then you have the foundation to build healthy relationships with others. When you are disconnected from yourself, you lose sight of your needs and begin to self-sacrifice, don't recognize your limits, and start to feel depleted and resentful.

The more you spend time with yourself in a reflective mindset, the clearer your needs will become. Another important part of your self-inquiry practice is exploring what gets in the way of setting aside time for yourself or expressing your needs and limits to others. Reflect on what feels difficult about asking for support, setting boundaries, or communicating directly. What are you worried will happen if you do? Have you had painful experiences of loss in the past? Your concerns are valid. Sometimes it makes others uncomfortable when you have needs or aren't as available to be an emotional support anymore. You may feel guilty about upsetting the other person or fearful of losing the relationship. There may also be other factors involved in how comfortable you are prioritizing yourself, such as cultural, gender, or family norms. Perhaps your immediate family has an indirect communication style and sweeps everything under the rug. Whatever you're feeling makes a lot of sense. These are important layers to explore during your self-reflection exercises.

Self-inquiry in the context of relationships is a tool for ensuring you know yourself well and are engaging in relationships that offer a sense of connection, fulfillment, and balance. The following two exercises will offer guidance for beginning to explore the state of your most important relationships and what changes you may want to make to improve those connections.

Reflecting on Your Relationship Needs

You have many types of relationships in your life, from close loved ones to acquaintances. For each of these relationships, you have different needs and capacities for connection. This journaling exercise will help you get clear on how your different relationship needs match up with reality and what changes you may need to make. For the following questions, answer for each of your significant relationships: parent, partner/spouse, best friend, family member, closest work colleague, and so forth.

How do you want to feel in your relationships?

Parent:

_____

_____

Partner/spouse:

_____

_____

Best friend:

_____

_____

Family member:

_____

_____

Colleague:

_____

_____

Other:

_____

_____

How much time do you want to engage per day or per week?

Parent:

_____

_____

Partner/spouse:

_____

_____

Best friend:

_____

_____

Family member:

_____

_____

Colleague:

_____

_____

Other:

_____

_____

What are your limits and boundaries?

Parent:

_____

_____

Partner/spouse:

_____

_____

Best friend:

_____

_____

Family member:

_____

_____

Colleague:

_____

_____

Other:

_____

_____

What do you need in this relationship to feel safe and supported?

Parent:

_____

_____

Partner/spouse:

_____

_____

Best friend:

_____

_____

Family member:

_____

_____

Colleague:

_____

_____

Other:

_____

_____

Reflect on what's working well in this relationship.

Parent:

_____

_____

Partner/spouse:

_____

_____

Best friend:

_____

_____

Family member:

_____

_____

Colleague:

_____

_____

Other:

_____

_____

Looking through your answers, take note of how you're currently feeling in your relationships and if something needs to change, such as setting firmer boundaries or asking for more support.

Relationship Inquiry

So often we set ourselves on autopilot and forget to check in on the state of our relationships. Over the next few weeks, write down all the people you spend the majority of your time with. Begin to notice your internal experience, whether or not your needs are getting met, and if there are any changes you wish to make to the amount of time you spend together.

Name:

How much time do you typically spend together per week?

Would you prefer to spend more or less time together?

When you're with this person, how do you typically feel (check all that apply)?

Happy	Grateful	Relaxed	Engaged
Sad	Optimistic	Agitated	Energized
Angry	Anxious	Stressed	Overwhelmed
Scared	Calm	Resentful	Exhausted
Annoyed	Distracted	Confused	_____
Safe	Focused	Distracted	_____

What other thoughts or physical sensations are you aware of when you spend time together?

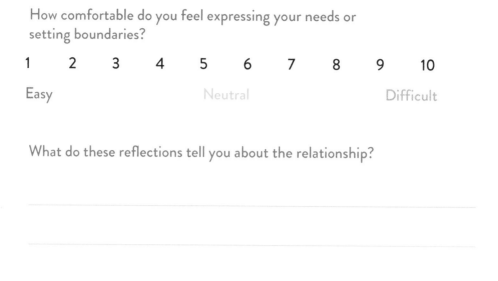

How comfortable do you feel expressing your needs or setting boundaries?

1   2   3   4   5   6   7   8   9   10

Easy   Neutral   Difficult

What do these reflections tell you about the relationship?

_____

_____

_____

Using the information you just gathered, you can begin to see how your relationships are impacting your emotional and physical well-being. It's important to regularly reflect on these questions to determine your need for boundaries and communication.

CREATING A SECURE RELATIONSHIP

As a licensed marriage and family therapist, I often get asked how to feel more securely attached and how to be a good communicator in relationships. My answer is always that you have to practice and try new ways of engaging with the people around you. There is only so much growth you can experience on your own, separate from others. When you engage in a relationship, you open another layer of awareness within yourself. This often brings up the communication template you learned from your immediate family (that you may not even have been aware of), the pain of losing people in your life through separation or death, and memories of feeling safe and understood by others. Being mindfully engaged in a relationship helps clarify how you want to feel, what your needs are, and how much you're willing to give of yourself. The practice of being mindful in relationships allows you to understand yourself and your needs more deeply.

Relationships invoke so many different emotions, including safety, security, grief, happiness, anger, or inspiration. Imagine a small toddler who is happy playing with their parent one moment, then angry that it's bedtime because they don't want to put their toys away, and then distraught when their parent leaves them with the babysitter. This is the nature of relationships: they can be a roller coaster of emotions that brings out your younger self who desperately wants to feel secure and safe. Often, the hardest part of relationships is their unpredictability: there's no guarantee you won't get hurt or lose someone. Mindfulness to the rescue! Of course, mindfulness can't make your relationships easy and risk-free, but the practice will soothe some of the emotional storm that happens when you feel triggered by someone. Practicing mindfulness also creates an opportunity for you to sit with your feelings without judgment and then to self-soothe when you are feeling triggered.

Being aware of and regulating your emotions may just be the most important skills you need for maintaining clear communication and strong connection. Think of a time when you were in an argument where you said something in anger, your emotions felt out of sync with the situation, or you were so overwhelmed with emotion that you had to flee the scene. You were most likely in fight-flight-freeze mode, with your emotions running the show. You may have been unaware at the time what the underlying trigger was to set off this reaction or how to soothe the emotional storm happening inside you. If this argument happened with a close friend, partner, or family member, you may have hoped they would step in to comfort you, even though you were also angry with them. It's all so confusing!

Fast-forward to the present when you are showing up to your mindfulness practice a little each day. This time, you notice the emotional storm in its early stages before the conflict gets out of hand. You're aware of your heart beating a little faster, your muscles tightening up, or your stomach churning. You realize that when your partner didn't respond to your bid for connection after you shared that you had a stressful day at work, it reminded you of being brushed off by your parent or caregiver when you would come home from school. This time, you notice the switch being activated, realize that your reaction is bigger than this particular moment, and choose to share the impact with your partner. Something like, "When you didn't respond to my day, it reminded me of my experience as a kid when I would feel ignored by my mom. Would you be willing to listen to more of my experience?" In this example, you're engaging your mindfulness muscle of observation of the present moment. You observe and share your observation of the other person's behavior without judgment (no response to the bid for connection), the impact (feeling ignored), and a need/request (to be listened to).

As you can see from this example, your personal mindfulness practice can have a great impact on how you engage in your relationships, transforming conflicts into dialogues. To achieve these benefits, it's important to continue building your informal and formal practice from the previous two chapters. The exercises offered in this chapter will add to that foundational practice, helping you stay in contact with yourself as you engage with others. Next, you will find an exercise to help you stay connected through gratitude, which research shows can increase relationship security.

Gratitude Exercise

Practicing gratitude increases connection and satisfaction in relationships (Algoe et al., 2010). When you feel connected to someone and appreciated by them, you are more likely to offer support and want to spend time together. Here are two ways to get you started on your own gratitude practice. You can practice at least once per week, either alone or with a loved one or friend.

Written:

1. Pick out a separate notebook just for your gratitude reflections. If you're doing this exercise with a partner, you can share the same notebook.

2. At the end of the day, take a few minutes to record what you are grateful for over the past week regarding the other person. Include qualities you appreciate and acts of service.

3. Take a few minutes to read over your reflections and glance back at a previous entry or two.

4. Pause to close your eyes and soak in the appreciation of the other person. Notice, without judgment, any thoughts, feelings, or sensations that are arising in you.

5. Slowly open your eyes.

Verbal:

1. Find a comfortable spot to sit facing your gratitude partner.

2. Take a few deep breaths together and sit quietly for a moment, reflecting on what you would like to share with your partner.

3. Take turns sharing what qualities you appreciate and acts of service you are grateful for from the past week regarding the other person.

4. After you each share, pause to close your eyes and soak in the appreciation of the other person. Notice, without judgment, any thoughts, feelings, or sensations that are arising in you.

5. Slowly open your eyes and thank your partner for practicing with you.

Noticing Bids for Connection

This exercise is geared toward noticing the needs of your partner or spouse, but this may also be useful for noticing indirect communication styles in family members, friends, and coworkers. A bid for connection could be verbal or nonverbal, but is often a subtle call for attention. Mindfulness can help you strengthen your relationships by keeping you aware enough of your surroundings to pick up on these easily missed cues. Here, I offer three ways to be more mindful of bids for connection.

1. Slow down to notice your partner during everyday interactions. How do they get your attention? What are they trying to communicate? If you're not sure what something means, check in with your partner. A sigh could either be a stress reliever that doesn't need any more attention, or a bid for support.

2. When your partner is sharing about their day or something they're interested in, such as an article or movie, slow down to listen and engage by reflecting what you hear, find out what were the best or most stressful parts, and ask questions to show you are interested in what they have to say.

3. If your partner initiates a hug, they may just want to connect briefly with you, or they may need more support. Take a moment to ask them how they're doing or if they need anything else.

These are just a few ways to bring mindfulness to your awareness of another's needs and subtle signals for connection.

CHAPTER REFLECTIONS

- ▸ The human brain responds to social disconnection in the same way it responds to physical pain.

- ▸ You can experience the benefits of meditation in your relationship whether you practice alone or with a loved one.

- ▸ Mindfulness strengthens relationship communication by creating space for empathy and compassion toward others while decreasing anger and emotional reactivity.

- ▸ Practicing mindfulness helps decrease stress levels and improve relationship satisfaction.

- ▸ Being aware of a significant other's bids for connection is an important component of relationship longevity and success.

04
Mindfulness at Work

You may not have considered bringing your mindfulness practice along to work with you because you don't have time during the day to slow down or can't imagine being able to drop into a meditative space. This is exactly why mindfulness can actually be your best tool. You need help mitigating the effects of stress throughout the day, detaching from being overly busy, and increasing awareness of your needs. Mindfulness is the path to finding a bit more work-life balance and decreasing the health implications of chronic stress. In this chapter, you'll discover common causes of stress in the workplace, see just how prevalent work stress is, and explore different tangible ways to be mindful at work.

BRINGING MINDFULNESS TO WORK

Work is such a defining part of our existence as human beings. When you meet someone new, what is the first question they typically ask you? Most likely, it's "What do you do?" Work has the potential to provide a sense of purpose or structure, typically fills the majority of our week, and allows us to financially support ourselves and our families. It's a vital part of our survival, yet it is often a source of stress. An astonishing 80 percent of people feel stressed at work (American Institute of Stress, n.d.), and the National Institute for Occupational Safety and Health reports 40 percent of workers feel extremely stressed, while 25 percent feel work is the biggest stressor in their lives (n.d.). According to the Centers for Disease Control and Prevention, mental health issues and stress affect work performance, engagement and productivity, communication, and overall functioning (2019).

What causes you the most stress at work or in relation to work? If you're not sure, you may have become so accustomed to correlating work with stress that it's hard to even distinguish the causes anymore. For many, work is stressful because there's no way to find work-life balance: working long hours without breaks or vacations has become the norm. Also problematic is ineffective leadership: supervisors either not providing adequate support and training, or going the other way by micromanaging everything you do. Of course, work is very stressful if you feel underpaid, have job insecurity, or work in an overstimulating or unpredictable environment, such as an open office, outside in the harsh elements, or in emergency services. Less talked about is doing work that makes you feel bored or disinterested. Even if you are paid well and have work-life balance and strong leadership, a lack of fulfillment at work can be just as stressful as being overwhelmed with too many responsibilities. Lastly, let's not forget the stress of not working if you need or want to be. That could be the most stressful situation of all.

Remember how you put mindfulness in your relationship toolbox in the last chapter? You can also add it to your work toolbox. Practicing mindfulness before or after work and on weekends is helpful, but you can also practice mindfulness *at* work to help you feel more calm and focused. A research review on the effects of practicing mindfulness-based stress reduction (MBSR) on employees' mental health showed a reduction in emotional exhaustion, burnout, and work stress; lower rates of depression and anxiety; more feelings of accomplishment and self-compassion; and improvements in sleep and the ability to relax (Janssen et al., 2018).

Incorporating mindfulness into your work routine not only helps your overall stress levels and mental health but also improves your work performance, focus, and ability to communicate clearly and build relationships with coworkers. It makes you more resilient and able to weather the storm during times of difficulty (Glomb et al., 2011).

At this point, are you loving all the benefits of practicing mindfulness at work, but skeptical that you'll actually fit it into your day? Who has time or space to meditate for 30 minutes on their lunch break, right? To figure out how to bring mindfulness to work, the clue is in the definition you read in chapter 1: mindfulness is the awareness that we experience when we pay attention, on purpose and without judgment, to the present moment (Kabat-Zinn, 2013). When you're at work, you can reap the benefits of mindfulness by simply slowing down and bringing awareness to your experience and what's happening around you.

Perhaps you start by sitting in your car or on a bench outside for a few minutes before you walk into work and taking a few deep breaths, checking in with yourself each time you go to the restroom, or using part of your lunch break to sit quietly with your thoughts and feelings. Of course, this is all easier said than done. Prioritizing your own well-being over the demands of work and letting go of the comparison with your coworkers may be challenging, but although it takes a bit of repetition and discipline, it does get easier over time. In the next section, you will have the opportunity to begin to explore a few specific mindfulness practices for the workplace.

SOOTHING STRESS AND INCREASING WORK PRODUCTIVITY

After reading about the high stress levels at work and the ways mindfulness can mitigate those stressors, you may be coming around to the idea of being more mindful at work. It's worth a shot, right? But what about *meditation* at work? This might feel like more of a stretch. Meditation is an internal practice that requires focus and uninterrupted concentration, which may feel pretty inaccessible at work, depending on the type of job you have. Thankfully, meditation can be practiced in many different ways and for various lengths of time. You don't necessarily need 30 minutes to sit quietly in the middle of your day. Let's be honest: Most people wouldn't be able to do that and actually have time to eat lunch, too.

Think of meditation at work not as your sole practice, but simply as an addition to your overall mindfulness practice. When your supervisor triggers you with a harsh bit of feedback, or your coworker talks over you in a meeting for the tenth time, you may become emotionally triggered. This response shuts down the prefrontal cortex of your brain, taking empathy, reasoning, and impulse control with it. Meditation can help you slow down, wring out your emotional sponge, recognize whatever emotions are coming up, and think clearly and communicate your thoughts without being reactive or impulsive. Saying something we didn't intend to say in our relationship is one thing, but taking our emotions out on our coworkers or boss can have a lasting impact on our livelihood.

To start conceptualizing what meditation at work could look like, begin by brainstorming spaces that you could use for meditation. As you go through your day this next week, look around for out-of-sight nooks or unoccupied spaces that provide respite from the noise and bustle around you. Depending on the setting, a few options could include a restroom, an outdoor space, your car, a stockroom, a conference room, or anywhere else you can take a few minutes to breathe without interruption. You may want to have a few spots tucked away in your back pocket in case one is being used when you need to step away to check in with yourself.

Once you have selected your space, you can select your practice based on how much time you have. If you literally only have one minute to pause, close your eyes to take your stimulation levels down and take a few deep breaths to engage your parasympathetic nervous system (the rest-and-digest system). If you have a few more minutes, take a scan of your body to notice any physical sensations, thoughts, or feelings. Whatever length of time you have to practice, approach your process without judgment, taking the stance of the impartial observer. You can model your meditation after the Simple Seated Meditation (page 8).

Don't forget that meditation doesn't always have to be a seated practice. You can also engage in a moving meditation, such as the Simple Walking

Meditation (page 17) or the Wringing Out Stress exercises (page 128), which may feel more supportive if you're sitting at a desk all day or want to incorporate meditative practices into your physical movements while working. You can start with the exercises shared at the end of this section or experiment with creating your own. You can fully engage with whatever activity you are doing by bringing your full attention to the process, whether it's painting a wall, entering numbers into a spreadsheet, mowing a lawn, or giving someone a massage. Simply slow down your actions, take note of the rhythm of your breath, and notice the quality of each movement. What are the internal sensations, thoughts, associations, and emotions as you move? Notice any textures, sounds, smells, or other sensory information as you do your work.

MINDFUL COFFEE BREAK

Getting up for coffee, water, or a snack is the perfect opportunity to engage your mindfulness muscle throughout the day. An audio recording of this meditation is available at AprilSnowConsulting.com/stress-workbook.

1. As you get up from your workspace, notice any physical sensations you're aware of, such as a stiff neck or sore lower back.

2. As you reach your destination, pause to take a deep breath and notice any thoughts or feelings you're aware of. Are you feeling hungry, thirsty, tired?

3. Slow down to observe the textures, tastes, and smells of your snack or drink as you consume it.

4. Intentionally return to your workspace, feeling your feet on the ground as you go.

This simple mindfulness exercise can be used multiple times per day to help you stay connected to your needs.

WORKDAY MORNING MEDITATION

You often hear how breakfast is the most important meal of the day; morning meditation could be the most important practice of your day. I equate it to filling up your tank and settling your nerves before embarking on a bumpy road trip. You can engage in this three-minute meditation in your car before you head into work, on the last few minutes of your train or bus ride, or at your desk before you turn on your computer. An audio recording of this meditation is available at AprilSnowConsulting.com/stress-workbook.

1.   Close your eyes and notice your body being supported by your chair.

2.   Feel your breath as it moves in and out.

3.   Imagine an empty container sitting beside you. Place any personal responsibilities or distractions inside the box, close the lid, then set it aside until the end of your day.

4.   Take a few more slow, deep breaths and welcome in a sense of spaciousness to be able to focus on your workday ahead.

5.   Set an intention for your day. What is the most important task to accomplish? Imagine how you'll feel when you check this off your to-do list.

6.   Slowly bring your awareness to your surroundings and open your eyes. You're ready to start work.

If you tend to hit the ground running in the mornings, try creating a daily morning ritual with this meditation to help you start your day with calm and intention.

LETTING GO OF COMPARISON AT WORK

Throughout your workday, there are so many opportunities to judge yourself, your coworkers, your job, your boss, and on and on. Most workplaces have some level of competition built in, causing you to constantly compare yourself and your performance to the person next to you, or even to others in your life, such as siblings or friends you grew up with. This mindset of comparison can create a lot of stress and anxiety if you feel like you aren't measuring up. It can also become very distracting, causing you to actually focus less on your work and the enjoyment of it, or it may begin to impact your overall sense of self-worth.

Getting stuck in a judgmental stance toward your coworkers or boss can also have a detrimental effect on your work performance and may cause conflicts in your relationships with them. Although people are typically the most critical of themselves, judging can also interfere with how they perceive others and their ability to build relationships, both personally and professionally. Releasing judgments will allow you to calm your reactivity and see others as they are, including their strengths and the many layers of their personality, helping you maintain a working relationship.

Judgment can push you to extremes of over- or underperforming. Underperforming looks like not applying to a job or promotion you really want because you don't believe you're as qualified as other candidates. Sometimes this thought could objectively be true, but often these limits are based purely on self-criticism. Overperforming looks like working long hours at the cost of your social life, personal relationships, family time, and overall health.

Getting stuck in a judgmental mindset may also cause you to look down on the job you do have, especially if you believe your occupation isn't valued by others or society at large. Before I started graduate school to become a psychotherapist, I worked in retail for many years. I felt self-conscious telling my new graduate school friends about my previous work history. If it wasn't for my experience training and mentoring others in my retail jobs, however, I never would have realized I wanted to be a therapist. If you can set down your judgments, whether coming from inside or outside of yourself, you can see the value and contribution of your work.

Whether you have a blue-collar service job or a white-collar office job or something in between, our society needs every job in order to function.

Letting go of judgment and comparison by taking the role of the impartial observer allows you to be fully present in your role, no matter what type of work you do. By stepping out of the vicious cycle of comparison and self-critique, you create an opportunity to take pride in your work, find meaning in what you do for a living, experience joy, and access creative solutions. One of my jobs during graduate school was at a very small natural foods store. After having worked at much more bustling stores before moving to the West Coast, I was so bored, and I felt insecure in my choice to take that job. I thought about quitting many times in the first few weeks, but then stepped back to see how I could make the most of the situation. I focused on connecting with the local customers and offering them support with their holistic health concerns, utilized my gift of organizing to create new inventory systems, and learned a lot in the process.

As you can see, judgments can become a barrier to feeling present and content, wherever you are in your work journey, and can damage working relationships. In the following exercises, you'll start to practice engaging with your coworkers without judgment and getting comfortable with imperfection.

Developing Better Relationships with Colleagues

When you work with someone, you only have the opportunity to see them from one side. Under the stressful conditions of a work environment, it's easy to have a fixed view of someone or make up your mind about their character or work ethic early on. When I worked in retail, I would often judge my coworkers who didn't have the same level of detail-orientation, and it interfered with me getting to know them as full people. When we make up our minds about someone before getting to know the full story, we completely cut off any chance to have a working relationship. In this exercise, I invite you to practice observing your coworkers (or boss) without judgment. Simply take note as you engage or see them throughout the day.

1.   What do you observe them doing? Perhaps getting coffee, making a phone call, helping a customer, or other activities that you do

as well. Without judgment or criticism, observe them moving throughout your shared space.

2.   Observe their physical appearance, again without judgment or comparison. What color hair do they have, how tall are they, and so forth? Notice any impulse to put qualifiers on your observations, such as "I wish I were as tall as they are" or "I don't like the way that shirt looks on them."

3.   Does this person remind you of anyone based on their behaviors, appearance, or speech? If so, does that explain your previous opinion of them?

4.   Are there needs you have in your interaction with this person that aren't getting met? How does that make you feel? What steps can you take to communicate these unmet needs in an effort to improve your working relationship? Take note of your experience from an objective stance.

Revisit this exercise anytime you notice yourself feeling judgmental or resentful toward your colleagues or when communication has become stalled.

Sitting with Imperfection

If you are judgmental of your coworkers, you are most likely even more critical of yourself. It's easy to take on a perfectionistic mindset, holding yourself to impossible standards at work. As a result, you may work long hours, sacrifice time with loved ones, skip lunch breaks, or work even when you're sick or need a mental health day. Mindfulness can help you practice non-judgment by accepting yourself and your environment as is. In this exercise, you will practice letting go of judgment and welcoming imperfection.

1.   Write down all tasks and responsibilities you could complete at work this week.

2.   Circle anything with a fixed deadline.

3. Transfer the circled items with deadlines onto a fresh, new
    to-do list.

4. Tuck the original list in your desk, filing cabinet, or someplace
    where you keep work documents out of sight.

5. Instead of staying late or sacrificing breaks to try to get everything
    done, focus only on essential items this week.

6. Notice what thoughts, feelings, or sensations arise throughout
    the week.

It can be helpful to revisit this exercise at the beginning of each week to
create a clear idea of your essential goals.

STAYING HEALTHY AT WORK

Recall that up to 80 percent of people feel some level of stress at work
according to the American Institute of Stress. In addition, 80 percent of medical appointments involve a stress-related component (Nerurkar et al., 2013).
With stress so common in the workplace, our physical and mental health are
at high risk. According to a World Health Organization study, depression and
anxiety alone led to one trillion dollars in lost productivity throughout the
world (Chisholm et al., 2016). On the flip side, practicing MBSR for even just
a few minutes a day (although 30 minutes is ideal) reduces and lowers the
recurrence of depression and anxiety (Hoge et al., 2017).

Think about your own experience of navigating stress at work and its
impact on your health. How often have you felt indigestion, anxiety, headaches, muscle tension, or other ailments as a result? Perhaps you're too
busy to even notice or check in with yourself throughout the workday.
Often the accumulating effects of stress at work go unnoticed, such as an
upset stomach that turns into an ulcer or anxiety that escalates to panic
attacks. Incorporating more mindfulness practices in general, not just at
work, will help you tune in and listen to the distress signals your body is
sending you before it's too late.

Many workplaces are so focused on output, comparison between
employees, and success that it's easy to completely forget that we are not
robots, but humans who need rest, reflection, connection, and nurturing

to survive and thrive. Due to this pressure to be perfectly productive, you may lose awareness of your physical needs and emotional state, and instead become overwhelmed by too many tasks, overstimulated by a noisy open office, or irritated by a supervisor who is disorganized or irresponsible. There are many stressors at work, any of which can lead to negative health consequences.

Another layer of attentiveness to your mind-body connection is awareness of your emotions and what triggers them in real time. Going into fight-flight-freeze mode in a conflict with a family member or significant other is one thing, but I'm sure you don't want to risk reaching that level of dysregulation at work. Entering fight-flight-freeze mode at work could look like forgetting your words in the middle of an important presentation, yelling at your boss, or sending an email impulsively that you later regret. As you build awareness of your experience in the workplace, you'll be able to course-correct these types of situations by engaging your mindfulness and self-regulation tools. You'll notice the signals, such as shallow breath or difficulty concentrating, that indicate you're reaching an elevated stress level and need a moment to calm down.

As you've begun to learn throughout this book, engaging mindfully gives you both awareness and control of your emotions so that you can show up as you need to at work. Mindfulness is not just about self-care and managing emotions: it can also help with decision-making and memory retention (Lazar et al., 2005) as well as increased focus and productivity (Good et al., 2015). In the following exercises, you can practice listening to your body's cues and engaging mindfully through movement.

Listening to Your Body

Work can take up so much of your focus and energy that you lose touch with your body. It's easy to skip lunch or forget to drink water, use caffeine to get you through the day or night, or take pain relievers to dull physical pain. These physical sensations, such as thirst, hunger, pain, or other ailments, are messengers that physical needs require attention. In this exercise, I encourage you to apply your mindful observation skills, without judgment, to your physical experience over the next week at work.

Check all that apply and record additional symptoms in the blank spaces provided.

Physical Symptoms

Headache	Wrist strain	Indigestion	_____
Eye strain	Sore feet	Stomach cramps	_____
Neck tension	Frequent colds or allergies	Fatigue	_____
Back pain or stiffness	Chronic body pain	_____	_____

Mental/Emotional Symptoms

Difficulty concentrating	Panic attacks	Hyperactivity	_____
Anxiety	Irritability	Feeling misunderstood	_____
Depression	Feeling overwhelmed	Disengagement	_____

Start to notice when you feel the symptoms you listed. Is it every day, around certain coworkers, or during particular projects?

_____

_____

_____

How often are you experiencing these symptoms? Daily? Weekly?

As you look over your reflections so far, what messages is your body trying to send to you?

Are there any adjustments you can make to decrease your stress levels, such as blocking off time for lunch or setting boundaries with a particular coworker who likes to interrupt you?

Use this exercise as a starting point to pay more attention to your body's cues throughout the workday. If you often skip lunch, forget to drink water, or experience physical and emotional stress symptoms, you may want to go through this exercise at the end of each week to see what adjustments you can make for your health.

Mindful Stretching

I know from personal experience that getting in touch with your body and giving attention to your emotional state can be uncomfortable at first. It's helpful to ease into this relationship with your body to notice what it's trying to tell you. An exercise that you may find helpful as a quick dose of self-care throughout the day is syncing your breath with movement. This practice is pretty subtle and can be done almost anywhere, with eyes open or closed depending on your needs. An audio recording of this exercise is available at AprilSnowConsulting.com/stress-workbook.

1. Take a moment to pause what you're doing.

2. Bring awareness to your breathing. Note the rhythm and location of your breath (shallow in your chest or deeper in your belly).

3. As you inhale, pull your shoulders up to your ears.

4. Hold for a count of one (or longer if that feels comfortable).

5. As you exhale, allow your shoulders to slowly roll down your back.

6. Repeat for three to five cycles, or until you notice yourself relax.

7. Pause for a moment to notice the rhythm and location of your breath now.

You can practice syncing your breath with any type of movement, such as raising and lowering your arms or stretching out your neck. Find what movement your body is asking for.

UNDERSTANDING YOUR NEEDS AT WORK

However you decide to incorporate mindfulness into your workday, whether using a formal seated meditation practice before work or an informal mindful activity during your day, self-inquiry will play a part. At the core of mindfulness is self-awareness and self-reflection, which help you observe what's happening inwardly and connect it to your external environment. This is especially important in relation to work, because during work it's easy and perhaps even encouraged to sacrifice your needs and lose connection with your experiences. As a result, it becomes nearly impossible to manage your stress levels and take care of your body.

So what does self-inquiry look like in the context of work? You're not necessarily going to break out your journal or have a deep, reflective conversation with a coworker during the day, although you may engage in these practices over a long lunch break. Whenever you practice any of the mindfulness exercises in this book, you will be engaged in some level of self-reflection, although there is room to be more intentional and bring self-inquiry to the forefront of your mindfulness practice.

A simple way to engage throughout the day would be to ask yourself, "How am I doing right now?" or "What do I really need in this moment?" The next time you reach for caffeine, chocolate, or some other type of comfort food, or you begin scrolling through social media on your phone, pause to ask yourself these two questions: How am I? What do I need? Maybe you're overstimulated by being on the computer all day and need a quick walk outside to feel the sun on your skin, or you're feeling irritated about a passive-aggressive comment a coworker just shared with you and need to call your friend for some support. Checking in with yourself throughout the day creates an opportunity to wring out that emotional sponge, calm your overstimulated nervous system, and make space for connection. Instead of your stress levels building because you're unaware of what's happening, you can redirect that momentum to your own self-care.

Now that we've explored the *how* of practicing self-inquiry, let's dive more into why this particular component of mindfulness work is beneficial. Taking time to check in with your overall well-being at work ensures you are in alignment with your values about the type of company you want to work for, the type of work that feels meaningful to you, and the types of coworkers you want to surround yourself with. Self-reflection practices also help create clarity around what goals you wish to pursue, how you want to feel while you're pursuing them, and what schedule actually feels sustainable. Lastly, taking time to reflect inward ensures that you stay in touch with your day-to-day experience to process any difficulties that arise, giving you more capacity for growth.

It's easy to get lost, caught up in the busyness and stress of work, and forget what would actually feel fulfilling and meaningful as a profession. What would your child self or teenage self say about the type of work you're doing if they could look at your life now? Would they feel excited, disappointed, or confused? How would you describe your current situation or how you arrived here? It can be helpful to pause and reflect on your life. There have been times when I wonder to myself, "How did I get here?" and "Did I actually choose this?" Then I realize that I made one decision that created a ripple effect. Sometimes this is a positive realization, and sometimes it may not be. In the following exercises, you'll get the opportunity to examine your relationship with work and reflect back on the dreams of your younger self.

Work-Life Balance Check-In

Often we are so busy trying to keep up with the expectations of work, family, and society that we forget to look at our inner world. Just as you take your car in for regular oil changes or go to the doctor for your annual physical exam, it's also important to schedule check-ins with yourself. Next are a few questions to help you explore your relationship with work and the changes you may want to make to decrease your stress levels and find more work-life balance.

When you think of going to work in the morning, what thoughts and feelings arise?

How do you feel throughout the day? When you arrive home?

_____

_____

_____

_____

What are the obstacles to prioritizing your needs at work?

_____

_____

_____

_____

What are the main stressors in your workplace?

_____

_____

_____

_____

How many sick or mental health days do you typically take per month?
Per year? How many would you take if you had an unlimited supply?

_____

_____

_____

_____

What mindfulness practices could you incorporate into your workday
to decrease stress levels?

_____

_____

_____

_____

Looking over your answers here will help you see what is causing you stress and where you can start to make changes. Return to this exercise at the beginning of each season or year.

Reconnecting to Your Dream Job

This exercise is meant to be completed after you explore the journaling prompts in the last exercise. Often a big source of work stress is not doing what feels meaningful or exciting, so this exercise will take you back to the work you've dreamed of doing throughout your life. An audio recording of this exercise is available at AprilSnowConsulting.com/stress-workbook.

1. Have a journal or notebook nearby for writing down your reflections afterward.

2. Find a comfortable seat where you can settle in without interruption for the next 10 to 15 minutes. If you're feeling alert, you may also lie down for this guided visualization.

3. Close your eyes and take a moment to feel your body being supported by the chair or ground underneath you.

4. Bring awareness to your breath and allow it to pull you further into your internal experience.

5. Take note and let go of any thoughts, feelings, or sensations you're aware of on your journey inward.

6. Travel back to when you were a small child. What did you really want to do for work when you grew up? What costumes or make believe did you enjoy the most?

7. What was exciting about that for you?

8. Move ahead to when you were in high school or college. What did you want to do for work then?

9. What was interesting about that for you?

10. If money were no object, what would you do for work now as an adult?

11. What draws you to that line of work?

12. Bring your awareness back to your breath as you slowly start to open your eyes.

13. Take a moment to observe your surroundings.

14. Write down any observations that surfaced during this visualization.

While the previous exercise focused on making adjustments to your current work, this exercise will help you see if there are any bigger career changes you want to make.

WEATHERING THE WORK STORM

Practicing mindfulness at work allows you to step outside the busy tornado of emails, phone calls, meetings, customer requests, or whatever else you are inundated with throughout the day. By bringing more attention to your daily experience, you begin to notice how work is impacting your physical, mental, and emotional health and why you may be having that experience. Essentially, mindfulness helps you create more self-awareness and weather that familiar storm of work stress. If incorporating mindfulness exercises and attention into your workday still seems inaccessible, that's completely understandable.

Due to your workplace's culture or leadership, it may seem off the table to create space for yourself or prioritize your self-care. Perhaps you don't want to tell your coworkers that you'd like to eat lunch alone or your boss that you aren't available to work late. I encourage you to stretch yourself in service of your well-being to see how you could care for yourself more. Even finding a few minutes of time for yourself during the workday could make a difference in your stress levels. Years ago a friend said to me, "You'll never hear a yes if you don't ask the question," and that has stuck with me ever since. Often there is more available to you than you realize, and sometimes the only obstacle is the fear of prioritizing your own needs. If you have no time to slow down, eat lunch, or set limits for yourself, there may be room to advocate for your needs at work without making any major changes. You may not be able to change jobs, choose a different schedule, reduce your hours per week, or work from home, but you can practice mindfulness to reduce the stressors at work and make it more sustainable over the long haul.

There is an abundance of opportunity to practice mindfulness informally at work, which you'll get to explore in the Mindful Workday Moment exercise at the end of this chapter (page 105). Anything you're doing at work can be approached mindfully. Simply give your undivided attention to the task in front of you, noticing your inner landscape and the sensory experience (such as sounds, smells, and visual observations) without judgment. Even if you are not able to increase break times or take a solo lunch, you can practice mindfulness without anyone even noticing. Some inconspicuous mindfulness exercises I like to practice when I'm feeling anxious in a meeting include pressing my feet into the ground, pushing my thumb into the palm of my hand for a subtle self-soothing massage, or even closing my eyes momentarily to take a few deep breaths.

In addition to informal practices, you may be able to incorporate modified formal practices if you have a bit more flexibility at work. You can do a quick body scan, take a few mindful breaths, do a short meditation, or go on a mindful walk to increase self-awareness and decrease stress levels. Remember that consistency is more important for stress reduction than how you practice or for how long (Lally et al., 2009).

This chapter offered many additional mindfulness exercises specific to your work toolbox that you can layer onto your MBSR foundation of seated and moving meditation. There are many options to choose from, so start with one that feels accessible right now and build from there. Over time, mindfulness will become a regular part of keeping you focused and calm during your workday.

Mindful Workday Moment

There are so many opportunities throughout the workday to slow down and integrate informal mindfulness. To refresh your memory, informal mindfulness is a practice of bringing your full attention to an everyday activity. For this exercise, choose any routine task that you frequently perform throughout the day, such as sweeping, making copies, or restocking inventory.

What task have you decided to practice mindfully?

To begin to bring more attention to this task, imagine yourself completing the task and list all the steps involved below.

_____

_____

_____

_____

For the next week, slow down to fully observe yourself while engaged in this task. What was the experience like for you?

_____

_____

_____

_____

Practice this exercise with different tasks to help you incorporate mindfulness into many areas of your work.

Mindful Lunch Break

One of the first questions I always ask my therapy clients who are stressed or anxious at work is, "Are you taking a lunch break?" Taking time for a proper lunch break can be difficult, but is absolutely essential to avoid feeling depleted and overwhelmed at the end of the day. I encourage you to not only take a lunch break, but also begin to insert some of your mindfulness practice into the routine, especially if you're struggling to find moments to pause throughout the rest of the day.

1. Set aside at least 15 to 20 minutes, 30 minutes if you can, in a quiet space such as your car, under a tree outside, or anywhere you can be away from the work crowd.

2. Put away your phone or any other distractions that may interrupt your focus.

3. Whether it's a sandwich, salad, or slice of pizza, take a moment to set out your food in front of you.

4. Pause to notice the colors, textures, smells, or any other observations of your meal.

5. Notice if you have any judgment about what you're eating and thoughts about what you should be doing instead of stopping for lunch. Observe and let go.

6. Take your first bite of food and allow it to linger in your mouth as you slowly chew.

7. What are the different flavors and textures? What is the temperature? Do these features change as you chew?

8. Continue to eat slowly, observing your experience along the way.

9. After you've finished your meal, stay seated for two to three minutes, allowing yourself to begin digesting your food before rushing back to work.

10. Reflect on the process of slowing down in the middle of the day to nourish and care for yourself. What was that like for you?

If you're an introvert, it's important to have quiet time during lunch breaks on most days. If you're an extrovert, you'll benefit more from more social lunches. Either way, try to have at least one Mindful Lunch Break per week.

CHAPTER REFLECTIONS

▸ When practiced regularly, mindfulness helps mitigate the effects of stress in the workplace, which impacts nearly 80 percent of the population.

▸ Practicing a few minutes of meditation at work, whether seated or moving, can help you manage your emotions, communicate more clearly with colleagues, and increase your focus and productivity.

▸ Comparison and judgment can be significant sources of stress and anxiety, leading to over- or underperforming in the workplace. Taking a mindful stance can help you see yourself, your colleagues, and your work environment more objectively.

▸ The pressures of work can lead you to ignore your body's messages regarding thirst, hunger, or rest, increasing the risk of physical illness or emotional burnout. A simple way of staying connected to your needs is to ask yourself "How am I?" and "What do I need?"

▸ No matter what profession you're in, mindfulness can be as simple as taking a few minutes before work to set an intention for yourself, slowing down to observe your inner experience as you move through the day, or carving out time after work to process your day.

05

Mindfulness and You

As you've seen throughout the book, mindfulness is a helpful tool in so many areas of life, but especially during times of stress. Unfortunately, your inner critic and emotional disconnection can get in the way of engaging in self-care. Cultivating a self-compassion practice can soothe the inner critic and help you accept your feelings, whereas mindful movement and yoga will wring out the physical effects of stress. As you'll discover in this chapter, mindfulness is the key to caring for yourself on all levels: physical, mental, emotional, and spiritual. The chapter concludes with guidance on how to design a mindful day in order to solidify your mindfulness practice in everyday life.

MINDFUL SELF-CARE

With all the stressors you encounter throughout any given day—at work, in your relationships, and inside yourself—managing it all can feel overwhelming. Ironically, the times when you need your mindfulness and self-care practice the most are often the times when it feels the most inaccessible. There never seems to be enough time in the day for self-care, you feel uncomfortable sitting quietly with yourself, your mind races when you try to go to sleep, or you feel guilty for prioritizing your needs over those of your family, friends, or work. There are so many barriers to self-care and committing to your mindfulness practice.

Take a moment to reflect and ask yourself, "How do I care for myself during times of stress?" It can be helpful to think about a recent example of when you were feeling stressed or overwhelmed. Maybe you had an argument with a family member because they didn't respect your boundaries, were worried about finances after some unexpected car repairs, or experienced a health scare during a routine checkup. What was your response to this stressor? Common responses are often comfort eating, avoiding talking about the problem, losing yourself in social media, retail therapy, or working overtime. Avoidance and distraction often exacerbate stressors over the long run and can take an emotional toll. It can be difficult to fully relax or focus when the stressor is looming in the background of your mind.

After reflecting on your typical responses to stress, think about how these responses impact you. Do they feel supportive and stress-relieving, or do they cause even more stress? If the latter is true, consider what changes you would like to make in your self-care practice. You can use the exercises in this book as inspiration.

During times of stress, mindfulness can help you sit with the uncomfortable feelings that may arise. However, mindfulness isn't only for mitigating stress in your life; it is also useful for engaging with yourself in deeply meaningful ways. It allows you to explore your inner landscape and what's most important to you, including how you want to show up in the world and what you want to do with your life. Although stress seems to be an unavoidable part of life, it is often worse when you are disconnected from your emotions, needs, and values. Mindfulness allows you to tune in and pay attention to what's happening along the way. You may notice stressors in their infancy stage, such as a small stomachache before it turns into an ulcer, increased fatigue and apathy before you are in a major depression, or disconnection in your relationship before you find yourself getting a divorce. Using mindfulness, you can become more aware of yourself and your surroundings to stop the buildup of stress before it piles up into a full-blown avalanche.

To keep stress levels low, incorporate some type of mindfulness practice on a daily basis. This will not only allow you to notice when stress is starting to accumulate, but you will also be able to regulate the emotional activation that occurs when you're going through the stress itself. Instead of ending up saturated and overwhelmed, you let go of a little bit of stress each time you bring awareness to your experience. During these instances of present-moment awareness, you have an opportunity to name what you're feeling, as well as process and release some of the emotional buildup and notice if your body needs anything. Sometimes when I'm in the middle of a long day at work, even just pausing to notice that I need a sip of water or a quick stretch can make a big difference. If I go through the day without breaks, I always feel exhausted, irritable, and overstimulated by the end of the day.

GETTING TO KNOW YOUR INNER VOICE

In our busy, tech-centered lives, there is less and less time for inner reflection. When I was growing up, I was with my thoughts all the time—riding in the car, waiting in line at the grocery store, or falling asleep at night. All those built-in pauses have now been replaced with screen time—checking social media or answering texts and emails. There never seems to be permission to unplug when so much is calling for your attention. Personally, I have to make a conscious effort to opt out of engaging with my phone. Often I intentionally leave my phone at home, turn it off, or put it out of sight so I am not distracted. It can be important to reflect on these questions:

▸ How often are you engaging with your phone when you could take a moment of silence instead?

▸ What's uncomfortable about sitting in silence?

▸ When you are sitting quietly, what internal narratives are you aware of?

Why is the lure of distraction so strong? Partly because there's a dopamine reward in our brains when we get a ping or a notification. More than that, though, there can be discomfort in the quiet moments. Sitting with your feelings is tough! That's why we love escaping reality so much. When you do get quiet, a flood of thoughts, feelings, and physical sensations surface, some of which you would rather avoid. The longer you avoid being with your internal experience, the louder the noise is when you finally stop and sit with it. I often ask my clients, "What gets in the way of taking care of yourself?" More often than not, there's an internal voice that says there's no time for self-care, that work or other obligations are more important, or that you're lazy, weak, or selfish for prioritizing your needs. Do any of these narratives sound familiar?

The inner voice that is full of opinions and loves to bully you into avoiding your needs is your inner critic. The inner critic often wants to protect you from failure, embarrassment, rejection, and disappointment, but it has a weird way of showing it. To get what it wants, the inner critic may use shame and guilt-tripping tactics, though many studies have shown that self-compassion is actually a more effective motivator than self-criticism (Breines & Chen, 2012). You'll learn more about self-compassion in the next section of this chapter. In case you get guilt and shame mixed up, like I used to: guilt is the feeling of "I've done something bad" (actions), whereas shame is a deeper feeling of "I am bad" (self). You may also recognize shame as feeling inferior, inadequate, or incompetent (Eddins, 2018).

An unchecked inner critic can limit your belief system, keeping you stuck in a place of fear and anxiety rather than confidence and abundance. You may not feel capable of pursuing your goals or taking risks to move your life forward in the direction you want to go. The next time you hear yourself regretting your actions or decisions, take a moment to pause and acknowledge the presence of your inner critic, and notice whether or not this voice sounds familiar. Often this negative self-talk is an internalized version of messages you heard in childhood, your community, or society at large. The way to defuse the inner critic's control over your mood, self-worth, and behavior is to catch it in action.

Although there are so many messages that tell you how you should live your life, many of those disregard the importance of self-care and the benefits of establishing a personal mindfulness practice. Meditation allows you to build a relationship with your inner voice, listen to your intuition, and be mindful that the critic is not left in charge. Otherwise, that inner critic can become so familiar that you forget that it's there, sabotaging your happiness and well-being. In the exercises that follow, you'll practice getting more comfortable sitting with silence and recognizing your inner critic. Remember to be patient with yourself as you begin to shift the presence of your inner critic. It took a lifetime to form this internal narrative, and it will take time for it to transform.

GETTING COMFORTABLE WITH SILENCE

Sitting quietly with yourself can be uncomfortable, especially if you haven't meditated in a while or are experiencing a higher level of stress in your life. This exercise provides a guide to ease you into spending quality time with your inner world.

1. Sit or lie in a comfortable position.

2. Set a timer for the length of time you intend to practice. Start with 30 seconds and increase as you feel comfortable.

3. Take a deep breath in through your nostrils and exhale through your mouth.

4. Gaze around your environment for a moment to orient you to the space, then slowly turn your attention inward, focusing on your breath moving in and out. If you get distracted, bring your awareness back to the breath, over and over again.

5. Briefly reflect on what this experience was like for you and rate the level of difficulty using the chart and rating scale provided.

Date of Practice	Practice Length	Difficulty Level*	Reflections (note here or in your journal)
	30 seconds		
	60 seconds		
	90 seconds		
	2 minutes		
	3 minutes		
	5 minutes		
	10 minutes		

1 = Easy (felt effortless, time passed quickly, could have sat for longer)

5 = Moderate (somewhat restless or distracted, but able to sit the whole time)

10 = Difficult (too uncomfortable physically or mentally, couldn't sit through the practice)

Slowly increase the amount of time you practice sitting silently. If the level of difficulty exceeds a 7, return to a shorter time until it reaches a 6 or lower.

IDENTIFYING YOUR INNER CRITIC

The first step to calming your inner critic is to notice that it's there in the first place and begin a dialogue with it. Often the critic goes undetected because it sounds just like your own voice. The next time you are under stress and notice yourself feeling anxious, fearful, guilty, or ashamed, take a moment to pause. An audio recording of this meditation is available at AprilSnowConsulting.com/stress-workbook.

1. Have your journal or a notebook close by.

2. Close your eyes and take a few deep breaths.

3. Zoom your attention in on your thoughts. What critical comments are you aware of?

4. Does this voice or the comments sound familiar? If so, who do they remind you of?

5. Slowly open your eyes and write down the critic's comments in your journal.

6. Imagine if you had a friend in the same situation you're in right now. What words of encouragement would you offer to them?

7. Compare the comments from the critic and your supportive comments to a friend. Which feel more helpful and motivating?

8. Take a moment to read the words of encouragement to yourself. Notice how you feel.

It's important to work with your inner critic often to shift it into a more self-compassionate tone of voice. Practice this exercise as often as possible until you feel the inner critic softening.

CULTIVATING SELF-COMPASSION

Now that you've started getting to know your inner critic, the next step is to begin replacing that constant chirp of judgment with a more compassionate voice. Self-compassion allows you to be with and accept whatever difficult experience you're going through. Instead of layering criticism, guilt, and shame on top of that struggle, you can identify the feelings that are coming up and gently validate how hard your experience is. You can also remind yourself that struggles are part of being human, and we often experience the same fears and hardships as others, such as loss, illness, financial instability, or not living life to the fullest.

Think about the last time you felt scared, exhausted, stressed out, or really worried about something. In that moment, which scenario would have felt more soothing and comforting?

1. Your friend comes over and tells you that you're fragile, too sensitive, or not trying hard enough, or that you just need to get over it.

2. Your friend comes over and listens to what you're going through without offering their opinion or giving advice. They softly say, "Of course you're feeling that way, anyone would be. It's going to be okay, I'm here for you."

In scenario number one, you start to feel even more down on yourself, perhaps moving even further into a dysregulated (fight-flight-freeze) state. In scenario number two, you feel safe with the comfort of your friend nearby. When you feel safe, you can start to process your feelings and eventually feel clearheaded enough to think about how you might move forward. Remember that when you're in fight-flight-freeze mode, you get stuck in your reptilian, impulsive brain, which cuts off your decision-making abilities.

This is the essence of the self-compassion practice. Self-compassion can simply be treating yourself as you would a good friend. You are replacing that inner critic with a friendly, supportive voice. You probably show your friends and family, even coworkers or neighbors, more kindness than you offer yourself. Take a moment to think about how many times a day you beat yourself up or push your limits. Would you ever want this for a friend? You would most likely encourage them to be more caring toward themselves and to honor their limitations.

A common concern about self-compassion is worry about losing motivation or becoming lazy or irresponsible. It may seem counterintuitive, but striving and criticism are not effective motivators. They don't increase happiness and in fact create more suffering. That inner critic may get some results from its bullying tactics, but you'll be acting out of fear and shame, not enthusiasm and meaning. This comes with an emotional cost over time, leading to insecurities, anxiety, and depression (Neff, 2015). As Christopher Germer, PhD, says in his book *The Mindful*

Path to Self-Compassion, "The more we wish our lives were different, the worse we feel" (Germer, 2009, p. 12).

Getting comfortable with self-compassion takes time, and it can be uncomfortable to treat yourself with care. You're often not encouraged to do so, you may not always have role models or support, or you may get criticized for being weak or lazy. It can also feel emotional to become aware of how little self-compassion there is in your life. When introducing this work to my clients, they almost always respond with initial resistance and grief when they recognize the lack of self-compassion or the lack of care and compassion from others present in their own lives. Give yourself time to settle into this practice: it's worth it!

Some of the benefits of practicing self-compassion regularly include:

- ▸ Increased ability to cope with stress (Allen & Leary, 2010)

- ▸ Increased job satisfaction and positive work engagement (Abaci & Arda, 2013; Babenko et al., 2019)

- ▸ Improvement of depression and elevated mood (Shapira & Mongrain, 2010)

- ▸ Decrease in anxiety after a stressful event and less avoidance of fearful situations (Allen & Leary, 2010)

- ▸ Lower rates of parental stress (Gouveia et al., 2016)

- ▸ Decrease in self-harm behaviors in adolescents (Jiang et al., 2016)

There are many ways to practice self-compassion, but generally you'll focus on being mindful of your present-moment experience, offering compassion and validation toward what you're feeling, and recognizing the shared experience of common humanity (Neff, 2015). In the following exercise, you'll have the opportunity to practice speaking to yourself more kindly during a difficult moment. Then, you'll expand that compassion outward to others in the Loving-Kindness Meditation (page 121).

Self-Compassion Practice

For this exercise, you can either write or speak the three parts of the practice. You can practice throughout the day, anywhere you are.

Self-Compassion Practice	Sounds or Looks Like . . .	Your Turn . . .
Mindfulness Take a moment to pause, notice your breath, and gaze inward. What thoughts, feelings, and sensations are present for you right now? What is the context of what you're feeling? Name that experience and what you're feeling without judgment.	*Ex: I'm feeling anxious because I have a presentation tomorrow.* *Ex: I'm feeling tired and scared after having an argument with my friend.* *Ex: I'm feeling frustrated with my body today.*	
Compassion + Validation In a kind and compassionate voice, as if you were speaking to a friend or a young child, offer yourself some validation for the difficulty you're experiencing.	*Ex: It's okay to feel anxious about things that are hard.* *Ex: Of course I'm feeling scared after having an argument with my friend. I don't want to lose them.* *Ex: When my body doesn't function the way I need it to, it's really difficult.*	
Common Experience To soften the inner critic or any shame that might be surfacing about how you're feeling, it's important to remember that you're not alone in feeling this way.	*Ex: I'm definitely not alone; lots of people get anxious before speaking in front of a crowd.* *Ex: It's so common to have arguments sometimes. There's nothing wrong with me.* *Ex: Everyone struggles with their bodies at some point.*	

After you've written or spoken the three components, it can be helpful to review the practice at least one more time while breathing slowly until you feel yourself begin to relax.

Loving-Kindness Meditation

Now you will take your self-compassion practice and offer that same compassion outward to others in the following meditation. A loving-kindness practice not only helps deepen self-compassion but can also reduce feelings of resentment and jealousy toward others (Stahl & Goldstein, 2019). An audio recording of this meditation is available at AprilSnowConsulting.com/stress-workbook.

1. Find a comfortable seat, close your eyes, and take a few moments to center yourself by focusing on your breathing.

2. Once you're settled in, close your eyes and bring to mind a memory of a time when you felt completely safe and accepted. Allow yourself to fully soak in the positive emotions of this experience.

3. Next, offer yourself three of these positive affirmations or create your own.

    May I be safe.
    May I be loved.
    May I be healthy.
    May I be strong.
    May I be peaceful.
    May I be hopeful.
    May I be grateful.
    May I be inspired.
    May I be _____

4. Take time to listen to the words and notice how you feel receiving this care.

5. Now bring into your imagination someone you really care about, such as a grandparent, child, mentor, partner, or best friend. Repeat three of these affirmations and imagine this person receiving the care you are sending to them.

    May you be safe.
    May you be loved.

May you be healthy.
May you be strong.
May you be peaceful.
May you be hopeful.
May you be grateful.
May you be inspired.
May you be _____

6. How did this experience differ from offering loving-kindness to yourself? Was it easier or more difficult?

7. You can stop here or continue on to offer loving-kindness affirmations to someone you feel mildly challenged by, such as a colleague or neighbor, and then outward even further to your entire community at once.

8. Sit quietly for a moment to notice the results of practicing loving-kindness toward yourself and others. Take a few deep breaths and slowly transition back into your day.

You may want to incorporate this Loving-Kindness Meditation into your weekly routine or practice it whenever you feel the need to offer yourself positive affirmations.

MINDFULNESS IN MOTION

Yoga prepares the body for meditation, although it can be a meditation in itself. In this section, we'll be exploring mindfulness in motion through hatha yoga and gentle stretching. Hatha yoga is a form of yoga that links physical postures with breathing. Yoga creates a bridge between the frenetic energy of stress and the calm energy of stillness. Translated from Sanskrit, "yoga" means "union" or "yoke," bringing together mind and body.

Yoga allows you to come home to your body and its innate wisdom. When you start listening to your body—your physical, emotional, mental, and spiritual needs as well as your intuition—you'll have the map to yourself and your life. You'll have access to your most powerful stress-reducing tool: your breath and the ability to calm your nervous system with a few simple movements. Yoga opens the door to reunite with your whole self. It wakes up the body and deepens your capacity for awareness.

Up to this point in the book, you have started to reconnect with your body through your breath and practicing the Body Scan Meditation (page 11). Now I'll invite you to take that awareness a bit further through mindful movement. This will allow you to feel even more embodied, or in your body, and in touch with your current stress levels.

Traditionally, mindfulness-based stress reduction (MBSR) uses the formal practice of hatha yoga to stretch, strengthen, and bring balance to the body (Kabat-Zinn, 2013). It is not about athleticism or flexibility, but about being present in your body and mind without judgment. While practicing, it's important to honor your body's limits and messages. If you have physical limitations, an injury, or a disability, that's okay. You can modify the practice to meet yourself where you are. That may change from day to day, so it's important to listen and pay attention to your body throughout the practice.

Instead of only focusing on what part of your body doesn't work the way you want, it's important to also see the parts of you that *do* work. As someone with chronic skin conditions, I can easily get frustrated when my skin is inflamed and itchy, especially if it limits my ability to move or show up the way I would like to. In these moments, I just want to hide in bed. Instead of skipping my practice altogether, I'll meet myself where I am: I either practice a few poses in bed or modify my practice to meet my body in the moment. Wherever you are is okay.

How often or how long should you practice? There were times when I thought I had to do a full yoga class or sequence to practice at all. When this time wasn't available or I didn't have the energy, I would skip my practice. I got stuck in an all-or-nothing mindset. As I got more familiar with the different yoga postures, I started experimenting with different lengths of practice. Now if I'm not able to commit to a full practice, I'll get on my mat for 10 to 15 minutes, or do a few poses after a stressful day to calm my nervous system. I've learned that a little goes a long way. Consistency is more important than length of time.

There are so many proven benefits to practicing mindful hatha yoga, including:

- ▸ Lower stress hormones such as cortisol (Katuri et al., 2016)

- ▸ Pain relief from headaches and backaches (Michalsen et al., 2005)

- ▸ Lower headache frequency and intensity (Kisan et al., 2014)

- Improved overall mental health (Smith et al., 2007)

- Improved sleep quality, including amount of time slept and ability to fall asleep (Manjunath & Telles, 2005)

- Significant decrease in anxiety levels (Javnbakht et al., 2009)

- Improvements in mood and decreased levels of depression (Woolery et al., 2004)

- Decreased levels of fatigue (Michalsen et al., 2005)

If you're committing to a full MBSR practice to establish your mindfulness routine, it is suggested to practice yoga 30 to 45 minutes at least three to four days per week, and the Body Scan Meditation (page 11) on other days (Kabat-Zinn, 2013). No matter what yoga postures you do or how long you are able to practice, the most important part of this formal meditation practice is mindfulness: paying attention to your body moment-to-moment without judgment and offering self-compassion for any limitations or emotions that surface.

In the exercises that follow, I offer two options for practicing mindfulness in motion, including my favorite yoga poses and stretches to help you feel calmer during times of stress.

Yoga for a Stressful Day

The yoga postures in this section are a collection of my favorite stress- and anxiety-relieving poses, which can be used as a full practice or done à la carte. Give yourself time to linger in each pose. Focus on your breath and your body's sensations, and make modifications as needed. As you move from one pose to the next, allow time for transitions. You'll find more yoga options in the Resources section at the back of this book (page 171).

Props needed:

- Yoga mat or blanket to lie on (you can also lie directly on the floor or on the ground if you're practicing outside)

- Folded towel or small blanket to put underneath your neck or hips

- Bolster or folded pillow to put under your knees

Modified Corpse Pose

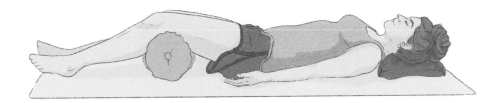

Spread out your mat or blanket and lie down flat on your back with arms and legs turned slightly outward. You can stay here, or place a folded towel or blanket underneath your neck and a bolster or folded pillow under your knees to support your low back. Relax here for two to three minutes at the beginning of your practice, or up to 10 minutes at the end. Focus on your breathing and notice any sensations in your body.

Reclining Mountain Pose

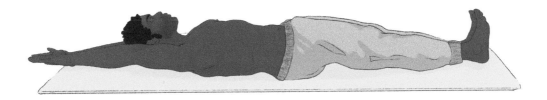

If you're using any blankets or bolsters, set those aside. Allow your arms to glide up overhead or as far as they will reach. Breathe in as you stretch your fingers and toes in opposite directions. Hold for just a moment, noticing where you feel the stretch. Breathe out and release the stretch, bringing your arms back down to your sides. Repeat a few times as desired.

Knees to Chest

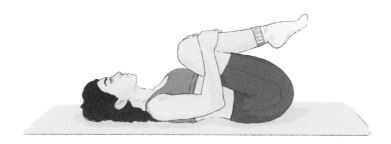

On your next exhale, bring your right knee up to your chest. Breathe in, then exhale and raise your left knee to your chest. You can gently hold both knees to your chest either with hands on the tops of the knees or underneath them. Check to make sure you're not holding tension in your neck. Give yourself a hug. Hold for about 30 seconds, or longer if that feels comfortable. As you exhale, release your hands and allow both feet to slide back down to the floor, keeping knees bent.

Revolved Stomach Pose

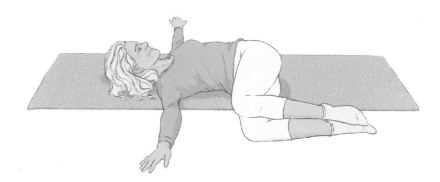

Stretch your arms straight out to your sides with your palms facing up to the ceiling. Exhale as you slowly bring your knees up to your chest and then over to your right side, creating a slight twist in your spine. Find the place where your neck feels most comfortable. Place your right hand on top of the knees or wherever it will reach. Left arm stays extended out to the side at shoulder height. Stay in this pose for one to two minutes, or until your body is ready to transition out. Repeat on the other side.

Child's Pose

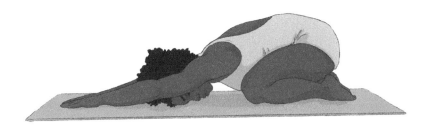

Come into a tabletop position on hands and knees. Check to make sure your knees are slightly wider than hip width and bring your big toes together. Take a slow, deep breath here, and as you exhale, allow your hips to sink back over your ankles. Your arms will stretch out in front of you, hands facing down and staying in contact with the mat. Make any adjustments to bring yourself into more ease in this pose. Rest here for up to three minutes, focusing on your breath and the sensations in your body.

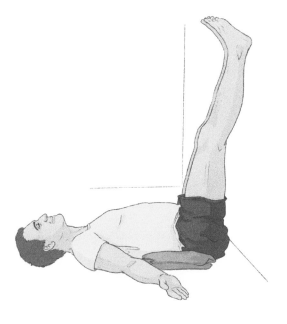

Legs Up the Wall

To get into this pose, rest your shoulder and hip against a blank wall with your legs extended out in front of you. Then swing your legs up to rest on the wall as your back comes to lie flat on the ground. Experiment with moving your hips closer to the wall and placing a folded blanket or towel under your hips to support your lower back. Your arms can stretch out to the side or rest on your belly. Support your neck with a folded towel or pillow if needed. Stay in this pose for about 5 to 15 minutes. When you feel ready to come out of the pose, bend your knees, push your hips away from the wall, and then roll over to one side. Take a few deep breaths and notice how your body feels before moving on.

Easy Pose

To finish your practice, or whenever you want to spend a bit of time in self-inquiry or meditation, find a comfortable seated position with legs crossed in front of you. Place a folded blanket or towel under your sitting bones to elevate your hips above your knees, which will relieve tension from your low back. Tuck your chin slightly in toward your chest and elongate your spine. Your hands can rest on your knees. Stay here as long as you like, focusing on your

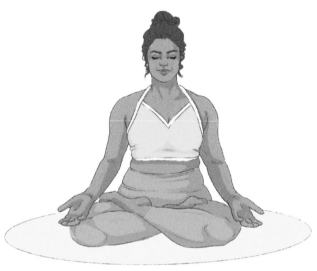

breath moving in and out. When you're ready to complete your practice, slowly open your eyes and look around your space before engaging in your next activity.

Wringing Out Stress

Use these stress-releasing exercises when you don't have the time or space to practice your yoga postures. These stretches can be done at work, sitting in your car, on a train, or wherever else you may be.

Shoulder Roll

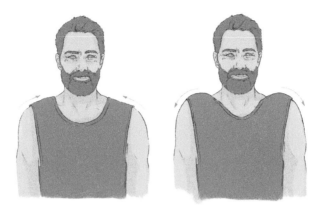

As you breathe in, scrunch your shoulders up toward your ears. Hold for a count of two, then roll your shoulders down and back as you slowly exhale. Repeat for three to five rounds or until you feel more relaxed.

Neck Roll

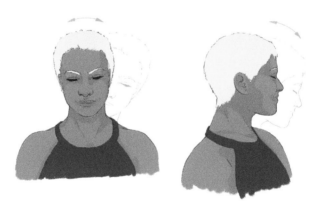

Take a slow deep breath in, and as you exhale, allow your neck to gently fall forward, bringing your chin closer to your chest. Breathe in and roll your neck to the right so that your right ear moves closer to your right shoulder. Exhale and allow your chin to come closer to your chest once again.

Breathe in and roll your neck to the left so that your left ear moves closer to your left shoulder. Repeat for one to three rounds or until you feel the exercise is complete.

Seated Spinal Twist

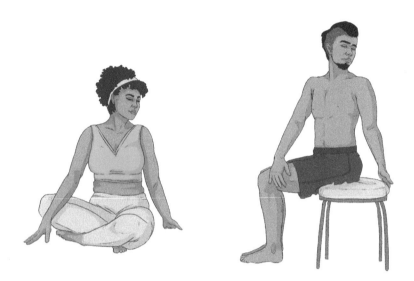

This pose can be done either seated in a chair or in Easy Pose (page 128). Breathe in and raise your arms overhead. Exhale as you twist slightly, bringing your arms down toward your left side and your gaze to look over your left shoulder. Take a few deep breaths here and then return to center. Repeat on the other side.

MINDFUL EMOTIONS

Emotions play an important role in your life by helping with decision-making, survival, and navigating relationships. Emotions also have a significant influence over your physical and mental state, yet they are often drowned out with distraction and avoidance through alcohol, drugs, shopping, social media, or comfort eating. What is your history with feeling your emotions? Does self-awareness come naturally to you, or do you avoid your emotions as much as possible? Perhaps one of the reasons you have gravitated toward mindfulness is to better understand the feelings you experience. It's natural to want to avoid feeling, especially when emotions are painful or overwhelming. Even positive emotions can be too much to digest sometimes.

Another factor that isn't discussed much outside of therapist circles is that multiple layers of feeling often occur simultaneously. Have you ever felt like you were feeling different emotions at the same time? For example, let's say you got offered a promotion at work. On the surface, this seems purely positive, right? You feel excited for the recognition and the opportunity to advance in your career. At the same time, you may also have imposter syndrome or begin to feel nervous about your new responsibilities, sad to stop working with your current coworkers, or stressed about all the work involved in transitioning out of one role and into another. That's a lot to sort through at once!

Another barrier to being with your feelings is that society encourages suppression and denial. Maybe you'll recognize some of these phrases: *get over it, suck it up, stop being so sensitive, you'll be fine, it's no big deal.* Notice how there are so many common expressions used to invalidate your feelings and encourage you to stuff them down. Unfortunately, feelings don't go away just because you aren't paying attention to them. They build up over time, causing the stress-related health concerns we discussed in chapter 1 (page 3) or spilling out without your consent.

You may experience unprocessed emotions overflowing into other areas of your life. It's very common to get angry at your boss and then take out your frustration at home instead by snapping at your partner or kids. Or the intensity of your emotions may feel out of sync with what's happening in the moment. For instance, you're watching a movie where the lead character loses their pet, and you can't stop crying hysterically. When your dog died last year, you told everyone you were fine. Instead of taking some time off to grieve, you put more energy into your work and did some retail therapy, hoping to distract yourself from feeling too sad. Watching the movie uncorked those feelings of sadness and loss that you thought you had avoided.

It's not always possible to feel your feelings in the moment. It can be too terrifying to recognize that you're in the eye of the storm. Instead, you focus on staying alive as your body moves into fight-flight-freeze mode. Often you have to get to safety before you can reflect on what you're feeling. When emotions pile up without any self-inquiry, they often compound into anger, depression, anxiety, and even physical health conditions. Thankfully, mindfulness can help you regulate your physical state and get you out of fight-flight-freeze mode, as well as bring awareness to what emotions are surfacing.

Being mindful of your emotional landscape may seem scary, overwhelming, or confusing at first. You may have a backlog of feelings to sort through. Be patient with yourself and lean on your self-compassion practice and other mindfulness tools. If you're struggling alone, it can be really helpful to reach out for support from a trusted friend, support group, or therapist. If you're unsure where to start, you can find a few options in the Resources section at the end of the book (page 171).

In the next exercises, you will have an opportunity to get more familiar with feeling your emotions.

Getting to Know Your Emotions

The first step in building a mindful relationship with your emotions is to create language around your feelings, and to know how your body typically communicates them, what thoughts are usually associated with them, and what circumstances are evoked. As you become more mindful of your internal landscape, you'll not only understand what the feeling is and how to recognize it by cues from your body, but also what tools help you manage it. Next, you'll see a sample feelings log and then one for you to complete. Copy this log into your journal, as it will be an ongoing reflection. I have listed the six basic emotions to get you started, but feel free to add additional rows as needed.

You can add to this Feelings Log after any of the mindfulness practices throughout the book. Notice how your emotional language and experience change over time as you spend more time in self-reflection.

Basic Emotion	Other Words or Phrases to Describe This Emotion	Thoughts That Arise While Having This Emotion
Fear	*Anxiety, nervousness, tension*	*I can't do this; I'm too scared*
Fear		
Surprise		
Disgust		
Sadness		
Happiness		
Acceptance		

Physical Sensations Associated with This Emotion	List Events or Circumstances When You Felt This Emotion	Helpful Tools or Other Reflections
Upset stomach, shaky voice	*Before a school presentation, walking alone at night*	*Deep breathing, yoga, and self-compassion really help*

Emotional Self-Inquiry

Once you start to create a language for your emotions, you can take your interaction with them a bit deeper to start a dialogue. The first step is to be mindful of the emotion and how deeply you're feeling it. Then, explore what comes up as a result of that emotion and move into self-soothing and regulation. It's helpful to practice acceptance without judgment and actively engage with your emotions. Over time, you'll have a map and a toolbox to navigate your emotions with more ease.

In this moment, I am feeling (write down whatever comes to mind):

_____

_____

_____

On a scale of 1 to 10, with 10 being the most intensely I've ever felt this feeling, I'm currently at a:

1   2   3   4   5   6   7   8   9   10

I know I'm feeling this way because (thoughts, sensations, circumstances):

_____

_____

_____

This feeling reminds me of (memories of past events):

_____

_____

If a good friend or loved one were here with me, I would want to hear these comforting words (offer self-compassion and validation):

_____

_____

_____

What I can offer to myself right now is (self-soothing and self-care):

_____

_____

Now that I have spent some time processing this emotion, the intensity level is currently at a:

1   2   3   4   5   6   7   8   9   10

Although you can practice this self-inquiry practice anytime, it will be especially informative whenever you're feeling stressed or having a heightened emotional experience.

MINDFUL DAY SELF-RETREAT

Experiencing a full day of mindfulness, or what I like to think of as a self-retreat, is a pivotal part of the MBSR curriculum and serves to solidify your practice. You will have the opportunity to integrate mindfulness into everyday activities at home. Unlike an overnight retreat, which is removed from daily life, engaging in mindfulness at home helps the practice stick. The real work of mindfulness is being able to cultivate awareness in the midst of everyday activities, as that is when you typically need the grounding and calming practices the most. Mindfulness, whether formal or informal, is usually practiced in chunks: 15 minutes of seated meditation here, 30 minutes of yoga there, a quick moment of presence while washing the dishes or folding the laundry. Making time for a mindful day creates a bridge between these islands of mindfulness to infuse awareness into every moment. The goal isn't necessarily to have a blissful experience, but to be present with whatever surfaces throughout an entire day.

Guidelines for Designing Your Mindful Day

▸ You can practice alone or invite others to join you.

▸ Clear your schedule for the day and unplug from any devices. Be sure to let others know ahead of time that you will be unavailable.

▸ Start your mindful day in the morning when you get up and practice until dinner, if possible. If a full day is not possible, try a half-day through lunch.

▸ For the yoga portion, you can practice any type of gentle, mindful yoga such as restorative, yin, integral, or Kripalu yoga. You can find online yoga options in the Resources section at the end of the book (page 171).

▸ Whatever practices you choose, slow down and focus on your experience in the moment, *paying particular attention to your:*

  · Sensory experience of sight, smell, taste, sound, and touch

  · Breathing

  · Inner world of thoughts, feelings, and sensations

▸ When you find yourself with space between practices, give yourself permission to be still. You can focus on your breathing, allow yourself to reflect on your experience of the day, or simply gaze around your environment.

Sample Mindful Day Schedule

Here you'll find an example of what a mindful day could look like, but feel free to design a schedule that works with your rhythms.

Time	Practice	Notes
8:00 a.m.	Mindful morning meditation + morning routine (shower, breakfast, etc.)	See Mindful Morning Meditation (page 25)
9:00 a.m.	Set your intention for the day	See Mindful Day Intention (page 141)
9:30 a.m.	Gentle yoga or mindful movement	See yoga options in the Resources section (page 171)
10:30 a.m.	Seated meditation	See Simple Seated Meditation (page 8)
11:00 a.m.	Self-inquiry through journaling or art	See Self-Reflective Journaling (page 42)
11:45 a.m.	Mindful walking	Outside or inside; see Simple Walking Meditation (page 17)
12:30 p.m.	Mindful cooking	See Mindful Cooking (page 37)
1:00 p.m.	Mindful lunch	See Simple Eating Meditation (page 18)
1:30 p.m.	Revisit your intention	Read through your journal entry from this morning to help you reconnect with your intention for the rest of the day
2:00 p.m.	Self-compassion or loving-kindness	See Self-Compassion Practice (page 120) or Loving-Kindness Meditation (page 121)

Time	Practice	Notes
2:30 p.m.	Mindful music or reading	Listen to instrumental or inspirational music; read poetry, sacred texts, or other inspirational material
3:00 p.m.	Mindful movement	Yoga, walking, dance, or another gentle movement of your choice
3:45 p.m.	Body scan	See Body Scan Meditation (page 11)
4:15 p.m.	Closing reflection	See Mindful Day Closing Reflection (page 142)

Designing Your Own Mindful Day

Using the blank schedule provided, design a mindful day schedule that fits your needs. Keep in mind that it's helpful to alternate sitting practices with movement practices to keep the body and mind from feeling fatigued or restless. You may want to pull from the exercises in this book to practice the various elements of mindfulness such as meditation, mind-body awareness, self-inquiry, and non-judgment. Feel free to incorporate your own exercises, too.

Time	Practice	Notes

Time	Practice	Notes

Mindful Day Intention

Before you begin your mindful day, take a few moments to set an intention to solidify why you're showing up and what you want to cultivate throughout your day. This intention is not about achieving a specific goal or being perfect, but instead bringing clarity to why you're showing up for yourself today. Let go of any specific outcome and focus more on your experience. An example of an intention could be to release judgment during your practice, or offer yourself loving-kindness when you feel stuck.

1. Grab a journal or notebook and pen, then find a comfortable seated position.

2. Close your eyes and take a few slow, deep breaths.

3. Allow your mind to wander to the end of your mindful day.

4. How will you feel after dedicating a day to mindfulness?

5. What will you do to get to this point? What will be nurtured within yourself today? Perhaps you invited in self-compassion and imperfection, allowed yourself to be with your feelings, or gave yourself permission to listen to your body's needs.

6.   Take a moment to quietly reflect with eyes closed and solidify your intention within yourself.

7.   Slowly begin to open your eyes and record your thoughts and feelings in your journal.

8.   Now you're ready to start your mindful day with intention and awareness.

You'll revisit this intention about halfway through your Mindful Day.

Mindful Day Closing Reflection

You practiced a whole day of mindfulness! Take a moment to offer yourself appreciation for practicing intentional self-care. This is not an easy task. Taking time to reflect on your mindful day will give you an opportunity to solidify your experience and notice your takeaways. You are welcome to practice this closing reflection by writing in your journal, or if your body is craving movement, head out for a silent walk to process your thoughts. If you practiced this day of mindfulness with a friend or family member, share your reflections with each other by practicing the Mindful Listening exercise (page 62).

1.   Start by reviewing your original intention for the day. Slowly read the words you wrote down this morning.

2.   Notice with curiosity what thoughts, feelings, sensations, or images arise as you reflect.

3.   What happened today as you expected? What was different?

4.   What was easier than expected? What was harder?

5.   How will you take what you learned today into your mindfulness practice?

6.   Take as long as you want to write in your journal, reflect, or share your experience with a friend.

7.   To close, take a few slow, deep breaths and offer yourself a loving-kindness affirmation: May I be_____.

CHAPTER REFLECTIONS

▸ Self-compassion is a more effective motivator than self-criticism. Other benefits of self-compassion include the increased ability to cope with stress, elevated mood, and decreases in anxiety and depression.

▸ Practicing yoga creates a union between body and mind, decreasing chronic pain, stress hormones, anxiety, and depression as well as improving sleep and overall mood.

▸ Emotions play an important role in many areas of life, such as decision-making and navigating relationships. Repressed emotions can lead to mental and physical health issues, but mindfulness can help you identify and regulate your feelings so they don't become overwhelming.

06

Going Deeper

As you go through the mindfulness exercises in this book, you may begin to uncover deeper emotional wounds and old memories, or your experiences might highlight current sources of stress that you haven't yet been able to process. All of this can make it uncomfortable or difficult to engage with your practice. In this chapter, you'll find guidance on how to practice mindfulness when life gets hard: sitting with your grief when you lose a loved one, job, home, or part of yourself; looking at struggles with self-esteem; using mindfulness to reduce the symptoms of chronic pain and illness; and exploring the common consequences of stress, such as anxiety, depression, and sleep issues.

WHEN THINGS ARE HARD

Mindfulness is often portrayed as blissful and effortless, but this just doesn't line up with reality. Life is messy and stressful a lot of the time. Your mindfulness practice will almost always overlap with something that feels difficult or imperfect, whether it's an unexpected stressor or difficult memory resurfacing. Admittedly, it can be uncomfortable to sit in awareness of your inner world during hard times. You may be practicing mindfulness during times of intense loss or betrayal, such as when you're diagnosed with an illness, laid off from your job, separated from a partner, losing a loved one, or struggling with a mental illness. When life feels overwhelming, you'll probably notice resistance to doing any type of mindfulness or meditation work, but this is when you need your practice the most.

There have been times when I cried through my meditation or yoga practice. Sometimes the reason was clear, such as after I lost my grandmother to lung cancer; other times I didn't know exactly why I was crying. As you deepen your practice, you may uncover old wounds or unresolved feelings from the past that have been stored in your body. Although it may feel uncomfortable in the moment, it's okay to allow these feelings to surface and pass through. You don't have to continue to allow them to take up space.

When you notice intense emotions or painful memories surfacing, name those feelings using whatever words feel right, and then validate them just as you did in the Self-Compassion Practice from the previous chapter (see page 120). If you become tearful, it's important to allow yourself to cry and process the emotions. You can assist by journaling in a stream-of-consciousness style. Make sure you continue to breathe and feel your body in your seat. When old wounds surface, it can be easy to travel back to when the memory was formed. If you start to dissociate—lose track of your surroundings—it can be helpful to orient yourself to your environment by noting in detail the colors, shapes, and textures you see around you.

You may be able to process your experiences on your own through self-inquiry, but if you're starting to feel overwhelmed or hopeless, I suggest reaching out to a therapist for a higher level of support; you can find more information in the Resources section in the back of this book (see page 171).

There won't always be words to describe the emotions released when you self-reflect, especially if these emotions were formed in the past, when you didn't have as many words or insights to describe your experience. Instead, you can lean on the language of your body: physical sensations or images that surface.

Throughout your practice, you may also be facing new difficult moments as well. Whether past or present, mindfulness can support you as you sit with the hard parts of life and look within. When life becomes overwhelming, mindfulness not only makes you aware of what emotions are surfacing, but it also helps you let go of judgment around those emotions. As we've discussed, although our culture is full of messages pushing you to avoid or minimize what you are feeling, mindfulness will help you bring acceptance without judgment while calming your rattled nervous system through breathing and grounding. Over time, you'll build up a resilience to emotional stressors, knowing how to intervene early before you completely shut down.

Even when you practice mindfulness every day and feel less stress overall, life will throw you unexpected curveballs that feel difficult to manage. At times like these, your mindfulness practice may feel different, but that doesn't mean you should stop. Continuing to show up for your mindfulness and meditation practice, even when things are hard, increases your tolerance to accept what is out of your control and process your feelings without judgment in the moment.

GRIEVING A SIGNIFICANT LOSS

One of the most stressful and universal experiences in life is grieving a loss. Grief is often associated with losing a loved one, but you may also feel it in other situations, like when a pet dies, your health or autonomy suddenly diminishes, or you lose your home to a fire. Much less talked about is the grief of losing parts of yourself as you enter a new stage of life or experience a stressful or traumatic event. This can happen when you become a parent, retire, or relocate to a new home. I often see adults who grieve the loss of a true childhood experience because they needed to take on an adult role at an early age or their caregivers weren't emotionally available. Essentially, any time you are separated from someone or something you care about, you may experience grief.

Just as there are many reasons to grieve, the grief response and process look different for each person. You will grieve in a way that is unique to you, and this may look different depending on how much time has passed and the type of loss. With grief comes a complex outpouring of emotions, such as anger, betrayal, deep sadness, anxiety, guilt, or regret. On top of this, you may also notice changes in your level of functioning or your overall health. Common reactions to a loss are difficulty sleeping or sleeping more than usual, changes in appetite, or temporarily losing interest in everyday activities. Other times, grief can spark an increase in activity, such as organizing paperwork and cleaning out closets, taking care of funeral arrangements, or scheduling medical treatments. Action can create a temporary sense of purpose and control, leading to feelings of safety. Mindfulness can help you notice your response to grief, whether it is more passive or active, and then offer yourself compassion.

The grieving process may not happen at the same time as the loss. When I lost my grandmother, I had the experience of anticipatory grief, as I knew my time with her was coming to a close. Anticipatory grief, or starting the grieving process before the loss, is also common when someone has been diagnosed with a life-threatening or chronic illness. Allow yourself time to ease into the mourning process leading up to and following a loss. Your first instinct may be to push away the intense feelings, as they are painful and overwhelming, but it's important to give yourself permission to be with your grief. Otherwise, the mourning process will be much longer and may create more complicated issues such as depression, inflammation, or a weakened immune system (Knowles et al., 2019).

You may worry that practicing mindfulness during times of grief will trap you under a flood of feelings. Although it may seem counterintuitive, the awareness that results from mindfully sitting with grief helps you identify and accept what you feel as you mourn (Kumar, 2005). Mindfulness can help you understand your feelings more deeply and keep in touch with what you need throughout the mourning process. It can also help you approach your process without judgment about how you should be grieving or how long it should take. Remember that grief is very individual, so give yourself permission to go at your own pace.

Grief comes in waves; it is not linear. You don't have to be with your difficult feelings all day to be actively mourning and moving toward acceptance of your loss. You are also allowed to have moments of feeling "normal": to laugh, connect, or experience levity if you can. Levity can be your life preserver through the messy storm of grief. By practicing mindfulness, you will create intentional moments to check in with your grief and be more equipped to ride the waves.

You can use any of the practices in this book as you're grieving. Here are two specific exercises to guide you.

SITTING WITH GRIEF

As difficult as it feels, it is important to be with your grief and any other emotions that come along with it. An audio recording of this meditation is available at AprilSnowConsulting.com/stress-workbook.

1. Find a comfortable position, either seated or lying down.

2. Place a hand on your belly as you slowly breathe in and out.

3. Allow your breath to guide you inward, noticing what physical sensations are present.

4. How and where is grief showing up in your body today? Maybe you feel numb, achy, tired, anxious, or heavy.

5. Place a hand where you feel the grief the most and offer yourself compassion: "I'm feeling _____ and that's okay. This is a hard time. Anyone in my situation would be feeling this way."

6. Take a deep breath in and as you exhale, allow your hand to fall back to your lap or wherever it's most comfortable.

7. Slowly open your eyes and gaze around your space.

If you have experienced a recent loss, return to this practice daily. Otherwise, you may want to sit with your grief on anniversaries of a loss or anytime a wave of grief washes over you.

CREATING A GRIEF RITUAL

Rituals provide a sense of purpose during times of loss, and studies have shown they lessen the negative effects of grief (Norton & Gino, 2014). Next, you will find three options to inspire your own ritual, but use your creativity to design one that feels right for you. Consider this exercise a meditation in motion to honor your loss, whether it's a person, place, part of yourself, or something else. Approach your ritual with purposeful attention and notice your inner experience without judgment as you move through it.

1. Select a space in your home to set up an altar. Adorn it with images, flowers, a candle, or other objects that remind you of your loved one or an earlier part of yourself. Sit at this altar each day to be with and honor your grief.

2. Listen to a song that helps you feel connected to your loved one, your true self, your culture, or a time in your life that you feel disconnected from. Close your eyes, take a few deep breaths, and then notice what thoughts, feelings, sensations, or images surface as you listen.

3. Visit a location that reminds you of the person you lost or the part of yourself that you are grieving. Sit quietly with the feelings that surface and offer yourself compassion.

You may want to create more than one grief ritual, depending on what feels right to you.

STRUGGLING WITH SELF-ESTEEM

There are many barriers to practicing mindfulness. One obstacle can be the hardest of all: self-esteem, particularly whether or not you can give yourself permission to take time for yourself.

A lack of confidence or self-worth can create a tendency to deny your own needs in order to please others, make it difficult to set boundaries to protect your time and energy, increase judgmental self-talk, and may lead to self-sabotaging behaviors such as substance use. Most people who struggle with this have experienced difficult childhood circumstances or stressful life events, or have internalized critical voices from caregivers or peers. If this is the case, you may have adopted an internal script that says your needs aren't valuable, real, or important. You may think you have to keep yourself small or bend over backward for others in order for them to like you. Often people who struggle with low self-esteem derive worth from what they do or what they can give to others, not who they are. This creates an unsustainable cycle of people-pleasing, self-sabotage, and burnout. It's a constant chase to fill up your esteem tank with external validation (instead of sourcing from within) or doing whatever you can to escape reality. As a result, you can become completely disconnected from yourself.

Many people struggle to feel worthwhile at some point in their lives, which makes it difficult to set aside time for a self-care routine. It's much easier to say yes to others than to yourself. As a result, you may notice resistance to doing something just for you. Your inner critic may jump in to criticize your choice to set aside time for mindfulness. This makes sense: the critic thinks you're putting yourself in danger by not following the usual script of doing for others, or that it's too risky to sit with those uncomfortable feelings. The critic fears that you'll lose relationships or confidence in yourself. Remind the critic that you're going to start caring for yourself and that although it may feel scary at first, you will feel better in the long run. Research has found that practicing mindfulness has a positive impact on self-esteem and life satisfaction (Pepping et al., 2013).

Getting stuck in people-pleasing mode or distracting yourself with work forms a barrier that blocks the clarity of your needs and wants. You become unable to see and feel the accumulating effects of stress on your body and emotional state. Focusing on the needs of others and escaping reality are quick fixes, but you often burn out quickly. Mindfulness serves as the bridge back to yourself. The path will be a little bumpy. Most likely a lot of inner judgment will surface, along with fear of being judged by others. As you've learned, a big component of mindfulness is unhooking yourself from that judgment to notice your experience objectively.

Often, folks with low self-esteem have a strong negativity bias: they miss the positive and zoom in on the negative, frequently blaming and shaming themselves in the process. With a steady mindfulness practice, you'll be more equipped to offer yourself compassion instead of criticism when negative thoughts or stressful experiences arise. Mindfulness helps you break out of the cycle of negative and judgmental thinking to become more attuned to your present-moment experience and able to see the good parts of yourself and your innate value, as well as acknowledge your accomplishments in real time.

Weekly Gratitude Practice

The best way to transform negative, judgmental thought patterns is to help your brain focus more on the positive moments. For this exercise, you'll write down at least three moments from the past week that you feel grateful for or that were positive experiences. A gratitude practice is most effective if it's consistent. I suggest finding a regular time to practice, such as Sunday evening before bed.

1. Take a moment to close your eyes and think about the past week: where you were, what you did, who you talked to, how you felt. Allow your mind to scan through without getting stuck on any one event.

2. When you come to an experience that felt positive or you feel grateful for, pause to record this event in your gratitude journal or a notebook. Record the moment in detail, making note of what was meaningful and how you felt.

3. Repeat the first two steps for at least three positive experiences, visualizing the moment in your mind and then writing about it in detail.

4. Notice if your brain wants to say "but" and then launch into what went wrong this past week or something you should feel bad about. Notice that impulse and bring your awareness back to your gratitude practice.

5.   Read through what you just wrote and allow it to sink further into your memory. Take a few deep breaths and notice how you feel at the end of this practice.

6.   Slowly transition into your next activity or bedtime routine.

Challenging Negative Thoughts

As you begin to focus more on the quality of your thoughts, you may be surprised to discover just how tough those negative beliefs are to get rid of. It takes time and practice to reframe negative thoughts into more well-rounded patterns. In this exercise, you'll start to track when a negative thought appears. Make note of what the circumstances are leading to the thought, what the thought is, and then transform it using a self-compassionate and validating tone. After some practice, this process will feel more natural and happen automatically.

Event That Sparked the Negative Thought	Negative Thought: What Would Your Critic Say?	Reframe: What Would a Good Friend Say to Offer Comfort?
Ex: I missed a deadline at work.	You're terrible at your job, and you're going to get fired.	It makes sense to feel upset. You're working really hard and have a lot on your plate right now.
Ex: Canceling plans to attend a friend's party at the last minute.	Everyone is going to be so mad at you for not showing up. What if they don't want to be your friend anymore?	It's okay if you are too tired to make it to the party. I understand, I've been there. Let's get together next week.

Incorporate this exercise into any self-inquiry or self-compassion practices that you are already engaged in.

NAVIGATING CHRONIC PAIN AND ILLNESS

As much as you mentally want to show up for your mindfulness practice, your body may become an unexpected obstacle. There are so many reasons you may feel uncomfortable being in your body mindfully, such as chronic pain, illness, exhaustion, body image, trauma, or gender dysphoria. Any of these reasons will make the process of paying attention more challenging, both physically and emotionally. No matter your relationship with your body, it's easy to take it for granted and ignore signals that it needs movement, nourishment, treatment, or rest. The more uncomfortable you feel in your body, the more you'll want to detach from it. Wanting to escape the discomfort in the moment makes sense, but unfortunately this can lead to more severe consequences later. The body is always sending you subtle messages to let you know what it needs, and the longer you ignore them, the more likely you are to experience more serious symptoms and stress-related health conditions down the road. Sometimes the body has to scream to get noticed, because most people only pay attention to their body when something is unavoidably wrong. For example, maybe you've fought through fatigue and a cold only to end up with bronchitis or an ear infection later. Or maybe you ignored an ache in your back, only to find out later that you have nerve damage.

Mindfulness allows you to see what may be contributing to or exacerbating physical conditions so you can make adjustments to care for yourself. For example, if you get chronic headaches, your instinct may be to disconnect from your body and distract yourself. What if instead, you put on your detective hat and became more aware of the circumstances surrounding these episodes? You may discover you get headaches when you work long hours at the computer, so you incorporate more breaks into your workdays to reduce your headache frequency. You won't always be able to completely avoid feeling physical discomfort, but mindful awareness could lead you to make helpful adjustments that bring you greater ease. Even if your physical symptoms stay exactly the same, your mood can be elevated by your mindfulness practice.

Let's be honest: when your body is not operating the way you want, it is stressful and exhausting. It's easy to feel like it will last forever. You may start catastrophizing, where you assume everything is falling apart. For instance, you tell yourself you're never going to feel okay ever again or that your pain will always be this intense. This tends to only cause more stress and anxiety, whereas staying mindful allows you to accept the present moment as it is, even if you feel your body is imperfect. Although it won't fix everything or make your pain go away completely, mindfulness can help reduce physical symptoms, lower stress levels, and calm the emotional storm that often happens on top of physical discomfort. Over the last 40 years, participants in the mindfulness-based stress reduction (MBSR) program at the University of Massachusetts Medical Center have reduced their physical and emotional symptoms by one-third after just eight weeks (Kabat-Zinn, 2013). Follow-up studies indicate even more hope, as participants continue to see improvements in symptoms for at least several years after the initial program, as most (90 percent) maintain their mindfulness practice (Kabat-Zinn, 2013). Changing the quality of your thoughts during meditation by unhooking from judgment and catastrophizing will ripple out into all the other parts of your body including how you respond to medications, the strength of your immune system, and your level of pain tolerance (Gardner-Nix, 2009).

Writing a Letter to Your Body

Whether you take your body for granted or you experience pain or discomfort on a regular basis, it's easy to forget how your body helps you every day. Take a moment to list all the ways your body is currently keeping you alive, such as breathing, pumping blood, or digesting food. Focus just on this moment and what you feel grateful for. Then write your body a letter to express gratitude for all it does, even in some challenging circumstances. See the sample letter on the following page for inspiration.

Dear Body,

Thank you for the many ways you support me. Even when the pain or discomfort feels so overwhelming, you continue to work to keep me alive. I often lose track of my breath, yet you keep me breathing. Sometimes I forget to eat lunch, but somehow you find fuel and remind me what I need. Even when I worry I'll never heal from a wound, you make magic happen. Thank you.

Love,

Me

Write your own letter here:

When you're experiencing symptoms or feeling stressed, reread your letter or write a new one to help you appreciate your body even when it is struggling.

Leaning into Discomfort

Although it may seem counterintuitive, being more mindful of pain or physical discomfort actually can help reduce the intensity of symptoms and decrease the emotional stress of what you are feeling in your body. In this exercise, you'll spend time listening to your body and tracking the impact of your mindfulness practice on your symptoms. An audio recording of this meditation is available at AprilSnowConsulting.com/stress-workbook.

1. Find a comfortable seated position, close your eyes for a moment, and briefly scan through your body from head to toe, taking a mental note of any physical sensations or discomfort you're experiencing in this moment.

2. Pause here to log your symptoms and intensity level in the chart provided.

3. Bring your attention to any part of your body that feels painful or uncomfortable. Take a moment to be curious about the discomfort, setting aside any worry about how long it will last or how you will fix it. Just notice the sensation with your full attention, maybe for the first time. What do you notice? Is your body sending you any messages right now?

4. Breathe into the pain or discomfort, sending healing energy and visualizing the pain dissolving away into the earth.

5. Slowly open your eyes and sit quietly for a moment, just you and your body.

6. Take a moment to note your symptom levels and journal about what came up for you during this exercise.

7. Slowly transition back into the rest of your day.

Date	Practice	Symptom	Intensity Level (Before Mindfulness)	Intensity Level (After Mindfulness)
6/21/2020	Body Scan	Back pain	7	6
6/22/2020	Body Scan	Back pain	7	5
6/23/2020	Body Scan	Back pain	6	4

1 = No Discomfort/Pain
5 = Moderate Discomfort/Pain
10 = Severe Discomfort/Pain

During times of heightened discomfort, it can be helpful to practice this mindful check-in at least once per day, depending on your needs.

MANAGING ANXIETY AND DEPRESSION

Perhaps one of the most common consequences of long-term stress on your mental health is experiencing some level of anxiety and/or depression. According to the National Institute of Mental Health, in the United States about 5.7 percent of adults experience generalized anxiety at some point, while 7.1 percent of adults suffer from at least one episode of major depression ("Generalized Anxiety Disorder," 2017; "Major Depression," 2019). To use a metaphor, think of anxiety as a squirrel, jumping around from place to place with nervous energy, whereas depression is a sloth, slow and sleepy. It's much harder to function in sloth mode than it is in squirrel mode, although both are dangerous to ignore.

Anxiety often shows up as excessive worry or fears about what may happen in the future, racing or looping thoughts, restlessness and agitation, difficulty concentrating, or an inability to fall or stay asleep. More severe cases of anxiety can manifest as panic attacks, obsessive-compulsive tendencies, or phobias, but for the purpose of this book I will focus on general anxiety, since this is more common. For most people, some level of anxiety is a part of life and shows up in mild forms of worry from time to time, but it doesn't cause any lasting distress. You might feel slightly anxious before an important work presentation or a first date, but those feelings of butterflies in your stomach quickly fade away. When you're feeling chronically stressed, anxiety tends to stick around and become less rooted in reality. You may begin to worry about everything and find it impossible to relax. This is because your nervous system has become overstimulated, which is common when you're stuck in worry mode for too long. It's like a computer you've run without restarting: eventually it starts to overheat, glitch, or even freeze up.

Depression is often sparked by a stressful life event that robs you of your confidence or stability, leading to feelings of defeat, loss, hopelessness, isolation, or unworthiness. As we discussed earlier in this chapter, unresolved grief is a common source of depression. As a result of these overwhelming stressors, you may start to notice sadness that doesn't easily go away, a sense of hopelessness, increased fatigue, irritability, loss of interest in things you used to easily enjoy, decreased concentration, negative thinking, poor self-esteem, or changes in appetite and sleep. A depressive episode can not only wipe out your energy levels and lower your mood, but can also significantly impact your body. As noted in the book *The Mindful Way through Depression*, 80 percent of people suffering from depression get medical treatment for mysterious aches and pains, which are actually the result of the body tensing in response to internal threats (Williams et al., 2007).

In both anxiety and depression, there's a loss of touch with the present moment. You get stuck worrying about the past or the future, have a distorted view of your reality, or experience uncomfortable physical symptoms that keep you from going inward. Under these conditions, it's easy to get swept away by negative thinking and start to believe there is something wrong with you for feeling this way. Mindfulness can bring you back to the present moment in order to take an objective, non-judgmental view of what's happening. You can break out of the cycle of critical and fear-based thoughts to offer yourself compassion and validation instead. As you do this, you'll be more capable of seeing the full picture of your reality, not just what's difficult. You can remind yourself of what led you here and why it makes sense to feel overwhelmed, sad, scared, exhausted, and so forth. Returning to your MBSR practice during hard times has been proven to greatly reduce anxiety and depressive symptoms for folks suffering from a wide range of physical and mental health conditions (Hofmann & Gomez, 2017). The practice also improves stress reactivity levels and coping (Hoge et al., 2013).

Quiz: Are You a Squirrel or a Sloth?

As you've seen and maybe personally experienced, symptoms of anxiety and depression can manifest differently in your body. If you're feeling more anxious and overstimulated, it's best to lean on mindfulness exercises that will be grounding and soothing. On the other hand, if you're feeling more depressed and lethargic, you may need more invigorating and movement-based exercises incorporated into your practice.

Are You a Sloth?

Shade in the bubble next to each statement that is true for you.

○ My thoughts feel sluggish or clouded.

○ I feel stressed.

○ I had a recent death or loss (e.g., relationship, job, home, pet, etc.).

○ I sleep a lot and have trouble getting out of bed.

○ I feel irritable and annoyed by people around me.

○ I don't think I'm good enough.

○ I have a low appetite.

○ I experience unusual aches and pains.

○ I want to do more, but I don't have the energy.

If you answered yes to at least three of the items on the Sloth list, try incorporating the following exercises from the book into your mindfulness practice:

▸ Simple Walking Meditation (page 17) or Body Scan Meditation (page 11)

▸ Mindful Self-Acceptance (page 63)

▸ Workday Morning Meditation (page 90)

▸ Identifying Your Inner Critic (page 116)

▸ Challenging Negative Thoughts (page 153)

Are You a Squirrel?

Shade in the bubble next to each statement that is true for you.

○ I worry about the future on a regular basis.

○ My brain won't shut off, especially when I sit still or try to go to sleep.

○ My body fidgets a lot.

○ I have difficulty focusing.

○ I have trouble falling or staying asleep at night.

○ I have had a panic attack in the last three months.

○ I worry about everything, all the time.

○ I feel stressed.

○ I want to do less, but it feels uncomfortable to slow down.

If you answered yes to at least three of the items on the Squirrel list, try incorporating the following exercises from the book into your mindfulness practice:

- ▸ Simple Breathing Meditation (page 16)

- ▸ Meditation for a Stressful Day (page 26)

- ▸ Sitting with Imperfection (page 93)

- ▸ Getting Comfortable with Silence (page 115)

- ▸ Yoga for a Stressful Day (page 124)

This quiz is for self-reflection purposes only. It is not intended as a substitute for treatment or assessment with a mental health professional.

Journaling for Emotional Release

It's easy to lose touch with reality during bouts of anxiety and depression. As a result, you may not notice that your emotions are beginning to build up and overwhelm you. Journaling can help you reorient to the present moment as you clear out your emotional backlog. Pull out your journal or a notebook and let the words spill out. Don't worry about punctuation or grammar; this is just for you. You can follow these prompts if you need help getting started.

I feel anxious when:

I feel sad when:

In my body, I feel:

Today I am grateful for:

_____

I will care for myself by:

_____

For support, I will reach out to:

_____

If your symptoms of anxiety and depression are interfering with daily functioning, such as sleep, appetite, or ability to focus, seek out the help of a licensed psychotherapist or psychiatrist. You can also consult with your primary care physician.

TENDING TO SLEEP ISSUES

What would a book on stress be without mentioning sleep? Though you need the most sleep during times of stress, it's often harder to come by. During stressful periods, people struggle with falling asleep, staying asleep, getting too much sleep, or having too little time for sleep. When feeling depressed, you could be getting too much sleep and feeling lethargic. On the other hand, if you're experiencing a sleep deficit, you may not be able to get to sleep at all due to insomnia, or you wake in the middle of the night because your mind is racing or because you have someone to care for, such as a new baby or an elderly family member. When I had shingles at age 32 during a particularly stressful period of my life, I had to take over-the-counter pain medication every three hours just to feel comfortable. This made it incredibly difficult to get enough rest, leaving me feeling irritable and even more tired throughout the day. There are so many stress-related circumstances that may impact your sleep.

Sleep deficiencies can impact your mood, causing increases in anxiety, depression, and irritability. You may also notice decreased energy levels, memory issues, and difficulty concentrating. Not getting enough sleep for extended periods can weaken your immune system, making you more susceptible to colds and increasing your risk for certain cancers, type 2 diabetes, and high blood pressure. Needless to say, sleep is essential, and unfortunately it's usually the first thing to go when you're under a lot of stress (Johns Hopkins Medicine, n.d.).

Even if you weren't aware of the far-reaching impacts sleep deficiencies can have, at some point you've probably experienced the frustration of not getting enough sleep. Paying attention to your sleep is an act of mindfulness and can give you important clues to your overall well-being. If you're not sleeping enough, or sleeping too much and waking up feeling lethargic, that's your cue to pay closer attention to what's going on around you. Is your busy lifestyle contributing to high stress levels or leaving little time for sleep? Perhaps you're drinking caffeine late in the day? Could there be underlying health issues, such as a thyroid condition? Are you a new mom with postpartum depression who could use some support? Whatever is happening in your world, take note of how it's impacting your ability to get a good night's sleep.

Trying to fall asleep can be so stressful. Often this is the only time of day where you are actually sitting quietly, not engaged with a screen or person calling for your attention. It's no wonder a flood of unprocessed thoughts, experiences, sensations, and worries from the day come flooding in, making it impossible to feel relaxed enough to drift off to sleep. Your body is like a small child, patiently waiting to tell you all about their day, but at this point you're too tired to listen. You can utilize mindfulness to improve your sleep in two ways. First, you can take those pauses throughout the day to listen to your body and reflect on your inner world of thoughts and feelings. Second, you can incorporate mindfulness into your bedtime routine to allow your body to access a relaxation response. In this mindful state, you'll be able to stay anchored in the present moment and let go of concerns about your to-do list, stop focusing on the stress happening around you, and worry less about whether or not you're getting enough sleep.

In the following exercises, you'll start to create a calming bedtime routine that will help you ease into bed and feel more relaxed.

Bedtime Routine Checklist

So often you may get into bed the moment you need or want to be asleep, but your body probably has other plans. It's important to create time for the transition between the waking and sleeping parts of your day. Your mind needs time to process the day and your body needs time to ease into relaxation mode. Having a bedtime routine can feel comforting and act as a signal for your brain that it's time to go to sleep. This checklist will help you create an intentional bedtime routine.

☐ Reserve your bed just for sleeping, so your brain doesn't think it's time to work when you really need to sleep.

☐ Shut off any screens, like laptops or phones, at least 30 minutes before you want to fall asleep.

☐ Get into bed at least 15 minutes before you need to fall asleep. If you want to read, meditate, or journal before going to sleep, give yourself more time.

☐ Start your bedtime routine at the same time each night.

☐ Intentionally set up your sleep space to be conducive to sleep, removing any unnecessary lights that keep you awake, using a weighted or heated blanket to help you relax, or adding a sound machine to block out street noise.

What else would you add to this checklist?

Once you have your bedtime routine in place, practice nightly for at least a few weeks until it becomes more automatic.

Simple Sleep Meditation

Often the biggest barrier to falling asleep is a busy mind that wants to ruminate or worry. The mind tends to pull you into the past or the future, making it feel impossible to relax enough to fall asleep. It can be helpful to pull your attention out of this thought spiral and back to the present moment, where you are safe and cozy in your bed. Start this meditation at least 30 minutes before you need to actually be asleep to get a full night's rest. An audio recording of this meditation is available at AprilSnowConsulting.com/stress-workbook.

1. Start by getting comfortable in your bed. Make sure your head feels properly supported, you have enough blankets to feel warm (but not too hot) and there are not any unnecessary lights or sounds bothering you.

2. If you haven't already, notice what thoughts and feelings are present from the day. Watch them float by like clouds in the sky, knowing that you don't have to do anything now; you are just observing.

3. Slowly bring your awareness to your breath, feeling it gently flow in and out. Imagine your breath nourishing you on the inhale and releasing tension from the day on the exhale.

4. Starting at the top of your head, consciously release tension from each part of your body. Breathe in, notice any sensations in that body part, and as you exhale, say, "May I be relaxed" or another affirmation that feels comforting.

5. When you finish scanning through your body, releasing tension as you go, feel your whole body relax into the bed. You are ready for sleep.

You may fall asleep during this meditation, but if not, give yourself time to fall asleep afterward by lying in the dark and focusing on your breathing.

MAINTAINING YOUR PRACTICE

As you come to the end of this book, you've had the opportunity to try out a wide variety of both formal and informal mindfulness practices, including breathing exercises, seated meditations, body scanning, yoga postures, self-compassion practices, and more. Allow me to refresh your memory on all the ways these practices can positively impact your physical and mental well-being when you engage in them on a regular basis. Mindfulness lowers stress levels by decreasing cortisol and other stress hormones as well as creating more resiliency to manage stressful moments when they arise. As a result, mindfulness has been shown to lower the occurrence of anxiety, depression, anger, fear, headaches, and chronic pain.

You'll notice the effects of mindfulness showing up in every area of your life, from how you talk to yourself to how you show up at work and in your relationships. Mindfulness strengthens your capacity for self-awareness and self-compassion while also creating more empathy and compassion toward others. This will help improve relationship communication and satisfaction, whether you practice alone or with loved ones. Your professional relationships will also receive the benefits of your practice, because you'll feel less work exhaustion or burnout and more focus and productivity while on the job. Since mindfulness has been shown to improve your ability to relax and decrease obsessive thinking, you might also notice that your sleep quality is better.

To experience these advantages, you need to devote as little as 10 minutes per day, although to maximize benefits studies have shown that 25 to 30 minutes of practice per day is most effective. It doesn't have to be perfect: skipping a day here or there doesn't remove the benefits. You can keep your practice simple and accessible, modeling it to fit your life and the types of practice you respond best to. For instance, I feel my best when I engage in 30 to 60 minutes of gentle yoga followed by 5 to 10 minutes of formal meditation, then journaling for a few moments. Perhaps you resonate more with mindful walking in the morning and seated meditation before bed, or some other variation. It's less about what you practice and more about consistency.

By now, you may have run into some challenges to practicing consistently, such as feeling distracted by your thoughts, being physically or emotionally uncomfortable, struggling to stay awake, or finding it difficult to set aside time for yourself. It can be helpful to remember that it's okay to show up as you are, busy mind or tired body and all. The most important part of mindfulness is showing up for yourself, over and over, with self-compassion and acceptance, free from judgment or thoughts of how you should be practicing. It will take time to feel at ease sitting quietly with yourself, but it does get easier. If needed, start with movement, guided, or short seated practices as you increase your tolerance. The best thing you can do for yourself is carve out a specific time and place in your home to practice. Over time, your body will come to expect to practice during that time.

CHAPTER REFLECTIONS

▸ Sitting in your feelings of grief and engaging in a personal ritual to honor your loss can help you move toward acceptance more quickly.

▸ Mindfulness positively impacts self-esteem and overall life satisfaction by breaking the cycle of negative thoughts and self-judgment.

▸ Just eight weeks of MBSR practice have been shown to reduce symptoms of chronic pain, illness, and a wide range of other physical and emotional symptoms.

▸ Anxiety and depression are common symptoms of stress. Mindfulness greatly reduces these symptoms while improving overall stress levels.

▸ Sleep disturbances can impact mood, energy levels, memory, and overall health, but mindfulness can help you engage the relaxation response you need to fall asleep.

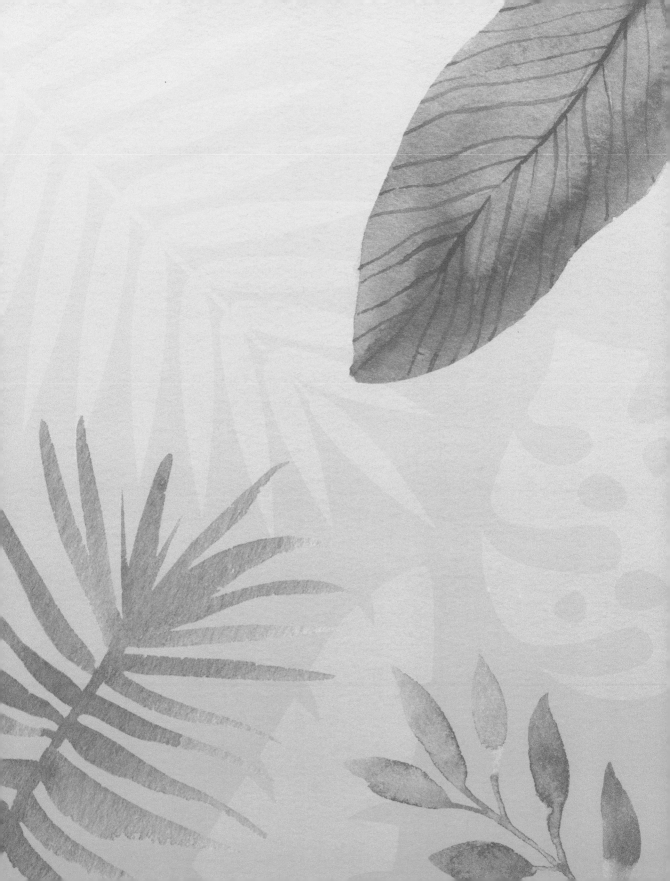

RESOURCES

Throughout this book, you have begun to form the foundation of your mindfulness practice, using mindfulness-based stress reduction (MBSR) techniques as the building blocks. When you are ready to deepen your practice, learn more about the MBSR program, or incorporate other modes of support, the resources in this section will help get you to the next level.

BOOKS

FULL CATASTROPHE LIVING: Using the Wisdom of Your Body and Mind to Face Stress, Pain, and Illness by Jon Kabat-Zinn. Dive deeply into the principles and practices of MBSR in this essential resource.

THE MINDFULNESS SOLUTION TO PAIN: Step-by-Step Techniques for Chronic Pain Management by Jackie Gardner-Nix. Learn specific mindfulness tools to change your perception of pain and reduce your symptoms.

THE MINDFUL WAY THROUGH DEPRESSION: Freeing Yourself from Chronic Unhappiness by Mark Williams, John Teasdale, Zindel Segal, and Jon Kabat-Zinn. Find helpful tools to break the cycle of self-blame and despair.

YOGA FOR EMOTIONAL BALANCE: Simple Practices to Help Relieve Anxiety and Depression by Bo Forbes. This book will guide you through restorative yoga and breathing practices to calm your stress levels.

MINDFULNESS-BASED STRESS REDUCTION (MBSR) PROGRAM

The UMass Memorial Center for Mindfulness at the University of Massachusetts offers in-person and online eight-week MBSR programs as well as free online meditations each week. Learn more at UMassMed.edu/CFM.

PSYCHOTHERAPY

If you're looking for additional support to help you manage your current stress levels or deeper wounds surfacing during your mindfulness practice, you may benefit from incorporating psychotherapy into your self-care. These directories will help you connect with a therapist in your area:

▶ Open Path Collective: OpenPathCollective.org

▶ Therapy Den: TherapyDen.com

SELF-COMPASSION

Guided meditations and exercises created by self-compassion expert and researcher Kristin Neff, PhD, can be found at Self-Compassion.org. I recommend starting with the five-minute self-compassion break.

YOGA

These websites offer gentle, online yoga classes that you can practice anytime or anywhere to decrease stress levels and soothe your nervous system.

▶ Kripalu Center for Yoga and Health: Kripalu.org

▶ Yoga International: YogaInternational.com

▶ Yoga with Adriene: YogawithAdriene.com

REFERENCES

Abaci, R., & Arda, D. (2013). Relationship between self-compassion and job satisfaction in white collar workers. *Social and Behavioral Sciences*, *106*, 2241–2247.

Algoe, S. B., Gable, S. L., & Maisel, N. C. (2010). It's the little things: Everyday gratitude as a booster shot for romantic relationships. *Personal Relationships*, *17*(2), 217–233.

Allen, A. B., & Leary, M. R. (2010). Self-compassion, stress, and coping. *Social and Personality Psychology Compass*, *4*(2), 107–118.

American Institute of Stress. (n.d.). *Workplace stress*. Retrieved from Stress.org/workplace-stress

Arlinghaus, K. R., & Johnston, C. A. (2018). The importance of creating habits and routine. *American Journal of Lifestyle Medicine*, *13*(2), 142–144.

Babenko, O., Mosewich, A. D., Lee, A., & Koppula, S. (2019). Association of physicians' self-compassion with work engagement, exhaustion, and professional life satisfaction. *Medical Sciences*, *7*(2), 29.

Breines, J. G., & Chen, S. (2012). Self-compassion increases self-improvement motivation. *Personality and Social Psychology Bulletin*, *38*(9), 1133–1143.

Brittle, Z. (2015, April 1). *Turn towards instead of away*. The Gottman Institute. Gottman.com/blog/turn-toward-instead-of-away

Carpenter, S. (2012, September). That gut feeling. *Monitor on Psychology*, *43*(8), 50. APA.org/monitor/2012/09/gut-feeling

Carson, J. W., Carson, K. M., Gil, K. M., & Baucom, D. H. (2004). Mindfulness-based relationship enhancement. *Behavior Therapy*, *35*(3), 471–494.

Centers for Disease Control and Prevention. (2019, April 10). *Mental health in the workplace*. CDC.gov/workplacehealthpromotion/tools-resources /workplace-health/mental-health/index.html

Chiesa, A., & Serretti, A. (2009). Mindfulness-based stress reduction for stress management in healthy people: A review and meta-analysis. *The Journal of Alternative and Complementary Medicine*, *15*(5), 593–600.

Chisholm, D., Sweeny, K., Sheehan, P., Rasmussen, B., Smit, F., Cuijpers, P., & Saxena, S. (2016). Scaling-up treatment of depression and anxiety: A global return on investment analysis. *The Lancet Psychiatry*, *3*(5), 415–424.

Choi, Y. M., Lee, D.-G., & Lee, H.-K. (2014). The effect of self-compassion on emotions when experiencing a sense of inferiority across comparison situations. *Procedia-Social and Behavioral Sciences*, *114*, 949–953.

Eddins, R. (2018, October 8). *Working with your inner critic*. Psych Central. PsychCentral.com/lib/working-with-your-inner-critic

Eisenberger, N. I., & Lieberman, M. D. (2004). Why rejection hurts: A common neural alarm system for physical and social pain. *Trends in Cognitive Sciences*, *8*(7), 294–300.

Gardner-Nix, J. (2009). *The mindfulness solution to pain: Step-by-step techniques for chronic pain management*. New Harbinger Publications.

Germer, C. K. (2009). *The mindful path to self-compassion: Freeing yourself from destructive thoughts and emotions*. The Guilford Press.

Glomb, T. M., Duffy, M. K., Bono, J. E. and Yang, T. (2011). Mindfulness at work. *Research in Personnel and Human Resources Management*, *30*, 115–157.

Good, D. J., Lyddy, C. J., Glomb, T. M., Bono, J. E., Brown, K. W., Duffy, M. K., Baer, R. A., Brewer, J. A., & Lazar, S. W. (2015). Contemplating mindfulness at work: An integrative review. *Journal of Management*, *42*(1), 114–142.

Gouveia, M. J., Carona, C., Canavarro, M. C., & Moreira, H. (2016). Self-compassion and dispositional mindfulness are associated with parenting styles and parenting stress: The mediating role of mindful parenting. *Mindfulness*, *7*(3), 700–712.

Harvard Medical School. (n.d.). *Now and zen: How mindfulness can change your brain and improve your health.* hr.Harvard.edu/files /humanresources/files/mindfulness_now_and_zen.pdf

Hofmann, S. G., & Gomez, A. F. (2017). Mindfulness-based interventions for anxiety and depression. *Psychiatric Clinics of North America, 40*(4), 739–749.

Hoge, E. A., Bui, E., Marques, L., Metcalf, C. A., Morris, L. K., Robinaugh, D. J., Worthington, J. J., Pollack, M. H. & Simon, N. M. (2013). Randomized controlled trial of mindfulness meditation for generalized anxiety disorder: Effects on anxiety and stress reactivity. *Journal of Clinical Psychiatry, 74*(8), 786–792.

Hoge, E. A., Bui, E., Palitz, S. A., Schwarz, N. R., Owens, M. E., Johnston, J. M., Pollack, M. H., & Simon, N. M. (2017). The effect of mindfulness meditation training on biological acute stress responses in generalized anxiety disorder. *Psychiatry Research, 262*, 328–332.

Holzel, B. K., Carmody, J., Vangel, M., Congleton, C., Yerramsetti, S. M., Gard, T., & Lazar, S. W. (2011). Mindfulness practice leads to increases in regional brain gray matter density. *Psychiatry Research, 191*(1), 36–43.

Janssen, M., Heerkens, Y., Kuijer, W., van der Heijden, B., & Engels, J. (2018). Effects of mindfulness-based stress reduction on employees' mental health: A systematic review. *PLoS ONE, 13*(1). DOI.org /10.1371/journal.pone.0191332

Javnbakht, M., Kenari, R. H., & Ghasemi, M. (2009). Effects of yoga on depression and anxiety of women. *Complementary Therapies in Clinical Practice, 15*(2), 102–104.

Jiang, Y., You, J., Hou, Y., Du, C., Lin, M.-P., Zheng, X., & Congfen, M. (2016). Buffering the effects of peer victimization on adolescent non-suicidal self-injury: The role of self-compassion and family cohesion. *Journal of Adolescence, 53*, 107–115.

Johns Hopkins Medicine. (n.d.). *The effects of sleep deprivation.* HopkinsMedicine.org/health/wellness-and-prevention/the-effects -of-sleep-deprivation

Kabat-Zinn, J. (2013). *Full catastrophe living: Using the wisdom of your body and mind to face stress, pain, and illness*. Bantam.

Kabat-Zinn, J., Lipworth, L., & Burney, R. (1985). The clinical use of mindfulness for the self-regulation of chronic pain. *Journal of Behavioral Medicine*, 8(2), 163–190.

Kabat-Zinn, J., Massion, A. O., Kristeller, J., Peterson, L. G., Fletcher, K., Pbert, L., Lenderking, W. R., & Santorelli, S. F. (1992). Effectiveness of a meditation-based stress reduction program in the treatment of anxiety disorders. *American Journal of Psychiatry*, 149(7), 936–943.

Katuri, K. K., Dasari, A. B., Kurapati, S., Vinnakota, N. R., Bollepalli, A. C., & Dhulipalla, R. (2016). Association of yoga practice and serum cortisol levels in chronic periodontitis patients with stress-related anxiety and depression. *Journal of International Society of Preventative & Community Dentistry*, 6(1), 7–14.

Kisan, R., Sujan, M., Adoor, M., Rao, R., Nalini, A., Kutty, B. M., Murthy, B. C., Raju, T., & Sathyaprabha, T. (2014). Effect of yoga on migraine: A comprehensive study using clinical profile and cardiac autonomic functions. *International Journal of Yoga*, 7(2), 126–132.

Knowles, L. M., Ruiz, J. M., & O'Connor, M.-F. (2019). A systematic review of the association between bereavement and biomarkers of immune function. *Psychosomatic Medicine*, 81(5), 415–433.

Kumar, S. M. (2005). *Grieving mindfully: A compassionate and spiritual guide to coping with loss*. New Harbinger Publications.

Lally, P., van Jaarsveld, C. H. M., Potts, H. W. W., & Wardle, J. (2009). How are habits formed: Modelling habit formation in the real world. *European Journal of Social Psychology*, 40, 998–1009.

Lazar, S. W., Kerr, C. E., Wasserman, R. H., Gray, J. R., Greve, D. N., Treadway, M. T., McGarvey, M., Quinn, B. T., Dusek, J. A., Benson, H., Rauch, S. L., Moore, C. I., & Fischl, B. (2005). Meditation experience is associated with increased cortical thickness. *NeuroReport*, 16(17), 1893–1897.

Manjunath, N. K., & Telles, S. (2005). Influence of yoga and Ayurveda on self-rated sleep in a geriatric population. *Indian Journal of Medical Research*, *121*(5), 683–690.

Michalsen, A., Grossman, P., Acil, A., Langhorst, J., Ludtke, R., Esch, T., Stefano, G. B., & Dobos, G. J. (2005). Rapid stress reduction and anxiolysis among distressed women as a consequence of a three-month intensive yoga program. *Medical Science Monitor*, *11*(12), 555–561.

National Institute for Occupational Safety and Health. (n.d.). *Stress at work*. CDC.gov/niosh/docs/99-101/pdfs/99-101.pdf?id=10.26616 /NIOSHPUB99101

National Institute of Mental Health. (2017, November). *Generalized anxiety disorder*. NIMH.NIH.gov/health/statistics/generalized-anxiety -disorder.shtml

National Institute of Mental Health. (2019, February). *Major depression*. NIMH.NIH.gov/health/statistics/major-depression.shtml

Neff, K. (2015). *Self-compassion: The proven power of being kind to yourself*. William Morrow Paperbacks.

Nerurkar, A., Bitton, A., Davis, R. B., Phillips, R. S., & Yeh, G. (2013). When physicians counsel about stress: Results of a national study. *JAMA Internal Medicine*, *173*(1), 76–77.

Norton, M. I., & Gino, F. (2014). Rituals alleviate grieving for loved ones, lovers, and lotteries. *Journal of Experimental Psychology*, *143*(1), 266–272.

Pepping, C. A., O'Donovan, A., & Davis, P. J. (2013). The positive effects of mindfulness on self-esteem. *The Journal of Positive Psychology*, *8*(5), 376–386.

Sevinc, G., Holzel, B. K., Hashmi, J., Greenberg, J., McCallister, A., Treadway, M., Schneider, M. L., Dusek, J. A., Carmody, J., & Lazar, S. W. (2018). Common and dissociable neural activity after mindfulness-based stress reduction and relaxation response programs. *Psychosomatic Medicine*, *80*(5), 439–451.

Shapira, L. B., & Mongrain, M. (2010). The benefits of self-compassion and optimism exercises for individuals vulnerable to depression. *The Journal of Positive Psychology, 5*(5), 377–389.

Smith, C., Hancock, H., Blake-Mortimer, J., & Eckert, K. (2007). A randomised comparative trial of yoga and relaxation to reduce stress and anxiety. *Complementary Therapies in Medicine, 15*(2), 77–83.

Stahl, B., & Goldstein, E. (2019). *A mindfulness-based stress reduction workbook*. New Harbinger Publications.

Tolahunase, M. R., Sagar, R., Faig, M., & Dada, R. (2018). Yoga- and meditation-based lifestyle intervention increases neuroplasticity and reduces severity of major depressive disorder: A randomized controlled trial. *Restorative Neurology and Neuroscience, 36*(3), 423–442.

Williams, M., Teasdale, J., Segal, Z., & Kabat-Zinn, J. (2007). *The mindful way through depression: Freeing yourself from chronic unhappiness.* The Guilford Press.

Woolery, A., Myers, H., Sternlieb, B., & Zeltzer, L. (2004). A yoga intervention for young adults with elevated symptoms of depression. *Alternative Therapies in Health and Medicine, 10*(2), 60–63.

Xu, M., Purdon, C. L., Seli, P., & Smilek, D. (2017). Mindfulness and mind wandering: The protective effects of brief meditation in anxious individuals. *Consciousness and Cognition, 51*, 157–165.

INDEX

ACKNOWLEDGMENTS

I want to express immense gratitude to my wife, Kate, for always being a loyal teammate and supporting my passions unconditionally. No matter what, you're always there to help me through to the end. Thank you for encouraging me to follow my dreams and take good care of myself along the way. This book wouldn't be possible without you.

To my first mindfulness teacher, my grandmother "Beebs," thank you for teaching me the importance of "being in the moment." From you, I learned the benefits of being present to what's unfolding in front of me and the value of connecting deeply with myself and those around me. You lead by example, meditating as a form of self-care and sharing your love of self-reflection with me. We have shared so many special moments together.

There have been so many spiritual teachers, mentors, therapists, and friends throughout my life who have helped me remain anchored to my internal experience and taught me there was a way inward. My relationship with mindfulness and this book are possible because of your wisdom and guidance.

Last, but not least, thank you to everyone behind the scenes who helped bring this book into the world. Specifically, my editors: Susan Lutfi who helped kick off the project, Katie Moore who went through the manuscript with a fine-toothed comb, and Vanessa Ta who supported me throughout the entire writing process.

ABOUT THE AUTHOR

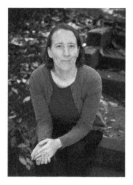

April Snow, LMFT, is a licensed psychotherapist and consultant in California who specializes in working with highly sensitive introverts, perfectionists, and high achievers to help them overcome the stress and anxiety of living in a busy, overwhelming world. A practitioner of meditation and yoga for more than 20 years, April has taught mindfulness workshops in various settings such as classrooms, retreats, and professional trainings. She regularly incorporates mindfulness-based stress reduction, self-compassion, and other evidence-based mindfulness tools into her clinical work. To learn more, visit AprilSnowConsulting.com.